NHA Phlebotomy Exam Prep +Anatomy and Physiology for Phlebotomist

Table of Contents

CHAPTER ONE: INTRODUCTION

"Proper preparation prevents poor performance" is a saying that is popular among students or anyone who has to undergo any form of assessment. Whether you're a seasoned medical professional or just starting your journey in the medical field, the fear of not being adequately prepared for an exam can be overwhelming. This is particularly true for students studying to become NHA-certified phlebotomy technicians.

The thought of taking such a comprehensive exam can be daunting, and the prospect of not passing can trigger fear if not altogether discouraging. Some of the questions participants on the journey to becoming certified phlebotomists have asked include, "How do I prepare for the NHA phlebotomy exam?", "Where do I begin?", "What should I watch for while preparing?" and "What should I expect in the exam?"

Preparing for the NHA phlebotomy exam requires more than just studying textbooks and attending lectures. Students need to understand the intricacies that surround an exam such as this, as well as how the exam has been presented to aspiring phlebotomists over the years. This will help them prepare to deal with the tricky questions the exams tend to present and will also put them at ease, boosting confidence all throughout the preparation phase.

The Purpose of this Book

In very simple terms, the purpose of this book is to guide the reader through acing the National Healthcareer Association (NHA's) Certified Phlebotomy Technician (CPT) exam. To achieve this, this book provides readers with a comprehensive review of the

CPT exam's content and structure, as well as practical tools and strategies for studying effectively.

This handbook is a study guide, not a textbook, and is therefore, not designed to provide comprehensive details about phlebotomy concepts. Although this book has been carefully designed and packed with the essential details any student will need to excel in the phlebotomy exam, it will not replace recommended training textbooks or given lecture notes in phlebotomy classes.

That said, it is important that every student who expects to succeed in the phlebotomy exam fully pay their dues by studying and going over materials to refresh their memories (especially if they've been out of school or active practice for a while), and finally, making use of this study guide.

Phlebotomy is a crucial skill in healthcare, and you will very well agree, considering the number of times the average person will experience a procedure involving phlebotomy in their lifetime! Despite how often phlebotomy procedures occur in medical facilities worldwide, it does not overrule the fact that it is a technique that requires a high degree of precision and expertise. This is why the NHA has provided the CPT exams to test the skills and knowledge of individuals who desire to become professional phlebotomists.

Due to the comprehensive nature of the exam, it can be a daunting challenge for students who are new to the field or lack practical experience. A well-designed study guide as this will help participants of the exam overcome these challenges by providing a clear roadmap for exam preparation and by offering practical advice for success.

One of the most important goals of this study guide is to provide the reader with a thorough understanding of the exam's content and structure. This includes an overview of the exam's format, including the number and types of questions, the time limit, and the passing score. The guide also covers the specific topics that are covered in the NHA phlebotomy exam. It will serve as a refresher for medical personnel who have long graduated from school and will also provide a rich supplementary study material for fresh students or graduates of phlebotomy lessons.

In addition to reviewing the exam's content and structure, this book includes a comprehensive series of practice questions that cut across the various topics explored, as well as provides detailed answers to these questions. While practicing these questions is highly crucial, the goal of this book is not just countless practice questions to keep students busy, but so that the student can identify areas of weakness they need to improve on and outline a clear roadmap for preparing for their exam. They can then revert to study resources and the chapters in this book to revisit those topics.

This study guide is also an excellent resource for a quick refresher as it helps candidates for the phlebotomy exam cut to the chase and bypass the information volume characteristic of phlebotomy textbooks. Here, they will find the most important details about each concept that the NHA's CPT exam focuses on.

In summary, this handbook serves as a productive and results-oriented guide that helps candidates become more knowledgeable about the concept of phlebotomy and passing the NHA's CPT exam. By the exam day, it is expected that everyone who has gone through this guide and has, of course, utilized all the helpful tips in it, will find 99% of the questions hassle-free and will have developed high confidence levels needed to be fully prepared to take the exam.

Overview of the NHA Phlebotomy Exam

The National Healthcareer Association (NHA) is a long-standing, widely recognized, and nationally accredited body that provides professional certifications in the field of healthcare. A certification from the NHA assures that the recipient is someone who is knowledgeable about their field and will be able to offer quality healthcare.

Because the NHA has demonstrated authority and expertise over the years, its certification has become one of the requirements most employers of healthcare professionals look for. The NHA offers eight healthcare certifications, of which the Phlebotomy Technician is one.

The NHA CPT exam is a rigorous assessment of a student's knowledge and skill in the field of phlebotomy. The exam covers an extensive range of topics, from anatomy and physiology to blood collection techniques, safety techniques, and patient care in the face of complications. Upon passing the exam, the participant earns a certificate that designates them fit to work in any healthcare facility as a phlebotomy technician.

The NHA CPT exam consists of just over 100 multiple choice questions plus 20 additional questions which candidates must answer before they begin the exam. The essence of the pretest questions is for the NHA to gather data. They do not count toward candidates' overall score in the exam.

The exam's comprehensive questions span across five essential topic areas in phlebotomy known as domains. Each domain is further divided into different subtopics classified as either knowledge statements or task statements. Knowledge statements include subtopics that candidates need to be educated about, while task statements refer to the processes that candidates must be able to know how to perform.

In other words, the NHA CPT exam encompasses both the theory and practical aspects of the field of phlebotomy. These ensure that students are critically tested for their all-round knowledge of the field and will ensure their overall success once they become certified phlebotomists or phlebotomy technicians.

Here is an overview of what each domain of the NHA CPT exam encompasses:

1. **Safety and Compliance:** This domain comprises 15 knowledge statements and 14 task statements. They all focus on safety precautions that must be maintained in phlebotomy to avoid health hazards to both the patient and the phlebotomy technician.

2. **Patient Preparation:** This domain covers the processes prior to the sample collection stage of phlebotomy, such as patient consultation and the determination of the collection site. It comprises 12 knowledge statements and 10 task statements.

3. **Routine Blood Collections:** This domain makes up a large portion of the examination as it tests the candidate's knowledge of the actual phlebotomy process up to the point where blood is withdrawn, and post-procedural patient care is offered. These are the typical day-to-day activities of a phlebotomy technician. The domain consists of 22 knowledge statements and 16 task statements.

4. **Special Collections:** This domain covers the rare and non-regular blood collection that can occur in patient care settings, such as blood collection for donation and peripheral blood smears. This domain is made up of 15 knowledge statements and 7 task statements.

5. **Processing:** The last domain has 8 knowledge statements and 7 task statements. It tests the candidate's knowledge of the steps involved after a blood specimen has been collected from patients.

Beyond these domains, the NHA CPT exam also incorporates a list of crucial knowledge and skills which are expected the exam candidates have honed. The knowledge of these skills is tested in how they are crafted in the questions featured in the exam. There are 16 of these core knowledge and skills:

1. Phlebotomy technicians' roles in laboratory testing

2. Phlebotomy technicians' roles in patient care

3. Medical terminologies used in the field

4. Blood components

5. Blood group systems

6. Aseptic techniques

7. Vascular anatomy as it relates to phlebotomy

8. The cardiovascular system

9. Hemostasis and blood coagulation

10. Needlestick Safety and Prevention Act

11. Pre-analytical errors and their impact on test results

12. Documentation and reporting in phlebotomy

13. Professionalism in phlebotomy

14. Verbal and non-verbal communication in phlebotomy

15. Patient characteristics and their impact on communication

16.   Ethical standards in the practice of phlebotomy

All these and the various concepts in the earlier outlined domains will be tested throughout the exam. The exam lasts two hours and can be taken online at schools and designated exam centers. Paper-based tests are also available in special situations. Within two days of taking the exam, candidates will get their results delivered to their individual accounts on the NHA exam portal, with their downloadable certificates if they pass.

Importance of Passing the Exam

Becoming a certified phlebotomist can open up a range of career opportunities in healthcare, including roles in hospitals, clinics, diagnostic labs, and other public health centers. It has been predicted that employment opportunities for phlebotomists and phlebotomist technicians will grow by 10% from 2012 to 2031. This is much faster than the average growth rate for jobs, with an average job opening of about 21,500 annually throughout the decade. [i]

Because blood analysis, withdrawal, and infusion remain essential parts of healthcare, there is no denying that phlebotomists and phlebotomist technicians will be in demand. However, no one can fully launch a career in phlebotomy unless they are certified by an accredited and recognized body such as the NHA.

Most employers look for the certification when employing phlebotomist technicians and phlebotomists as it demonstrates to employers and patients that they have the necessary knowledge and skills to perform phlebotomy procedures safely and effectively.

In addition, sitting for the CPT exam and passing can boost confidence and passion in the field, propelling participants to achieve their career goals faster and setting them on course for what would be an exciting career in phlebotomy. Passing the exam indicates candidates' knowledge of the act of phlebotomy, their preparation to step into the field, and their wholesome understanding of performing phlebotomy in order to contribute meaningfully to the quality of patient health and safety.

Nevertheless, a previous record of failure in the NHA phlebotomy exam is not the end of the world. After all, successful people are known for their ability to fail forward and learn from their past mistakes. Should the reader be sitting for the CPT exam for a second time, taking hold of this study guide is an excellent and laudable step in the right direction. As already mentioned, this study guide will expose participants to their weak points and help them identify what they need to do better. The first chapter is a great way to start, as it emphasizes what phlebotomy is and how important it is to healthcare – an indication that choosing to earn a certification in the field is a wonderful opportunity to save lives as a healthcare professional.

CHAPTER SUMMARY

- This book provides the most important details about each concept that the NHA's CPT exam focuses on.
- The National Healthcareer Association (NHA) is a long-standing, widely recognized, and nationally accredited body that provides professional certifications in the field of healthcare.
- The NHA exam covers the following domains:
  - Safety and Compliance
  - Patient Preparation
  - Routine Blood collections
  - Special collections
  - Processing
- Each of these domains are well covered in this book.

- Becoming a certified phlebotomist can open up a range of career opportunities in healthcare, including roles in hospitals, clinics, diagnostic labs, and other public health centers.

CHAPTER TWO: RELEVANT ANATOMY AND PHYSIOLOGY

"No Knowledge Can Be More Satisfactory to A Man Than That of His Own Frame, Its Parts, Their Functions, And Actions." - Thomas Jefferson

The human body can be divided into regions for the sake of description. It can be divided into upper limbs, lower limbs, head and neck, thorax and abdomen, pelvis, and perineum. The body systems also include the digestive system, gastrointestinal system, circulatory system, musculoskeletal system, respiratory system, endocrine system, nervous and reproductive systems. All these systems work together to coordinate processes necessary for life.

However, for the purpose of this book, the focus will be on the circulatory system and related structures because this system is closely related to phlebotomy.

The Circulatory system

The human body comprises millions of cells that need nutrients to survive. These cells receive nutrients through effective digestion, breakdown, and transportation mechanisms via the circulatory system. The circulatory system delivers nutrients, hormones, and oxygen to cells across the body. It also removes waste products, such as Carbon (IV) oxide, from the body. It comprises blood, blood vessels, and the heart.

The heart is a tough, muscular organ that serves as a pump for the entire body. It pumps deoxygenated (with low oxygen content) blood from the body to the lungs, where it is then oxygenated. It pumps oxygenated blood (with high oxygen content) back around the body.

To perform its function, the heart is divided into four major chambers. These chambers are:

- The right atrium/auricle, which receives deoxygenated blood from the superior and inferior vena cava.

- The right ventricle, which receives blood from the right atrium.

- The left atrium/auricle, which receives blood from the pulmonary vein coming from the lungs; and

- The left ventricle that pumps blood into the aorta and from there to the rest of the body.

Pulmonary circulation is responsible for the oxygenation of blood. In this circulation, blood flows from the right ventricle to the lungs, where oxygenation occurs, and then back to the left atrium.

Systemic circulation takes the oxygenated blood from the left ventricle to other body parts.

A valve separates the right atrium from the right ventricle, known as the tricuspid valve. It prevents the backflow of blood, ensuring a unidirectional blood flow. The bicuspid or mitral valve is located in the left chamber between the left atrium and ventricle. It also prevents the backflow of blood, ensuring a unidirectional flow of blood.

The heart is composed of 3 distinct layers:

- Endocardium: The inner lining of the heart.

- Myocardium: The middle layer that is contractile in nature.

- Epicardium: This refers to the outermost layer of the heart that is fibrous and contains the coronary arteries.

The Blood Vessels

The blood vessels include the aorta, arteries, arterioles, capillaries, venules, veins, superior vena cava, and inferior vena cava.

These all form the path of blood flow through the body and can be broadly put into arterial supply and venous drainage of the body.

Overview of the Venous Drainage of the Body

Blood moves in one direction, all veins carry blood to the heart, and all arteries carry blood away from the heart. All arteries (except the pulmonary artery) carry oxygenated blood, while all veins (except the pulmonary veins) carry deoxygenated blood.

Veins all carry deoxygenated blood (except the pulmonary vein) from different body parts to the heart.

Generally, veins carry blood from all the body's tissues, cells, and organs back to the heart. They are in different sizes, ranging from very large veins that run parallel with their similarly named arteries to unnamed tiny veins that form an irregular and collateral network with the large veins.

Veins can be classified based on their positions. They can be:

Superficial veins: These are situated right under the skin, just below the fatty layer. They are the ones most suitable for venipuncture. Examples of superficial veins in the lower limb include the great and small saphenous veins, which both arise from the dorsal venous arch of the foot. The great saphenous vein, after running its course, drains into the femoral vein directly, while the small saphenous vein eventually drains into the popliteal vein. Examples in the upper limb include the cephalic and basilic veins.

Deep veins: Deep veins are situated deep in the muscles and course along bones. Examples in the upper limb are the brachial, axillary, subclavian, anterior and posterior interosseous, radial, and ulnar veins. Deep veins in the lower limb include the anterior and posterior tibial vein, the fibular vein, the popliteal vein, the femoral vein, and the external iliac vein.

Connecting veins: Connecting veins are short intermediary veins that connect the superficial and deep veins. Deep veins transport blood from cells, tissues, and organs to the heart. Since blood flow in the venous system is from the tissues to the heart, blood flow is usually sluggish. But there are some mechanisms that the venous system works with to propel blood towards the heart and prevent a backflow of blood.

Muscular compression: Since deep veins are usually situated around muscles, the muscles around help to squeeze those veins so that blood is moved back to the heart. A typical example is the calf muscles and the deep veins in the leg whenever a person steps. Veins can be easily compressed because they have thinner and larger lumen walls than arteries. They are easily distensible and can accommodate more blood. In fact, between sixty to seventy percent (60 -70%) of blood volume is found in the veins. Therefore, muscle compression is a very important way of maintaining blood flow in the body.

Valves: Another adaptation that veins have is the possession of valves. These valves close and open in one direction to allow only a unidirectional blood flow in veins toward the heart.

The upper and lower limbs are the most important regions in phlebotomy, and it is important to understand the relevant anatomy, especially concerning blood flow. There are veins at the surface of the upper limb, which usually begin at the dorsum of the hand, called the dorsal venous network. From there, these veins unite to form the cephalic and basilic veins, which ascend the upper arm.

Just before reaching the elbow, the cephalic vein connects with the median cubital vein, which passes diagonally across the anterior aspect of the elbow. The basilic vein ascends, traversing the medial end of the dorsal venous network of the hand. It eventually enters deep into the brachial fascia and forms the axillary vein.

In between the cephalic and basilic veins is a median antebrachial vein, which starts at the base of the dorsum of the hand and ascends to occupy the space between the cephalic and basilic veins. This vein is quite variable in different bodies.

Overview of the Arterial Supply of the Body

Arteries transport blood away from the heart. Arteries generally transport oxygenated blood from the heart to the tissues, except for the pulmonary artery. The pulmonary artery transports deoxygenated blood (blood with low oxygen content) from the heart to the lungs. They usually run deep with the deep veins.

Arteries do not need valves like the veins because they directly receive supply from the heart, and the blood flowing through them is at relatively high pressure. Their walls are also not as thin and compressible as that of the veins.

Arteries have a wall that comprises 3 major layers:

- Tunica intima, which is the endothelium or inner layer.

- Tunica media: Refers to the smooth muscle present in the arteries and gets to expand or contract as needed.

- Tunica externa is the outer layer, and it communicates with other tissues and structures.

Blood flows under high pressure from the heart into the aorta, which then forms the aortic arch, which gives off 3 branches that supply the head and part of the upper limb. They are the brachiocephalic trunk (largest), left common carotid artery, and the left subclavian artery.

From the aortic arch, the blood continues as the descending thoracic aorta. Here it gives 2 classes of branches: the visceral and the parietal branches, which give rise to other arteries. The thoracic aorta continues as the abdominal aorta, which gives rise to the celiac trunk, the superior and inferior mesenteric artery, the renal arteries, and the iliac arteries.

The arteries of the upper limbs are the subclavian artery, axillary artery, brachial artery, radial artery, and ulnar artery.

The arteries of the lower limb are the femoral artery, profunda femoris artery, popliteal artery, dorsalis pedis, posterior tibial artery, and fibular artery.

Selecting a Site for Phlebotomy

In selecting a site for phlebotomy, the veins that are situated in the antecubital fossa are the most preferred. They are usually easily accessible and wide enough to accommodate the needle. They are also not as close to other delicate structures like nerves or arteries, which are usually deep.

The veins that are preferred in order of choice include the following:

- Median cubital vein
- Cephalic vein
- Basilic vein
- Dorsal venous network
- Foot

In choosing phlebotomy sites, some of the veins to avoid include:

- Sclerosed veins: These types of veins are hard or cordlike in nature. They are seen in some disease conditions or patients taking chemotherapy.
- Tortuous veins: these veins are not straight and can make the process of obtaining the sample difficult. They are also very prone to infection and can produce altered or incorrect results.
- Arm with IV fluid running: the fluid would affect the results of the tests.
- A−V fistula site: Avoid arteriovenous fistulas. The test results would be inaccurate, and the fistula could also be affected.

- In diabetic patients, the foot should be avoided because of the increased risk of diabetic foot disease. But generally speaking, phlebotomists would only use the foot as a last resort.
- Areas of burns should also be avoided.
- Infected portions of the skin should be avoided.
- Upper extremity ipsilateral side of a mastectomy: Specimens taken from this side can be affected by lymphedema, which would alter the results.

CHAPTER SUMMARY

- The circulatory system delivers nutrients, hormones, and oxygen to cells across the body. It also removes waste products, such as carbon dioxide, from the body. It comprises blood, blood vessels, and the heart.

- The heart is a tough muscular organ that serves as a pump for the entire body. To perform its function, the heart is divided into four major chambers:

    i. The right atrium/auricle
    ii. The right ventricle
    iii. The left atrium/auricle
    iv. The left ventricle

- Pulmonary circulation is responsible for the oxygenation of blood.

- Systemic circulation takes the oxygenated blood from the left ventricle to other body parts.

- The heart is composed of 3 distinct layers:
    a. Endocardium: The inner lining of the heart.
    b. Myocardium: The middle layer that is contractile in nature.
    c. Epicardium: This refers to the outermost layer of the heart that is fibrous and contains the coronary arteries.

- The blood vessels include the aorta, arteries, arterioles, capillaries, venules, veins, superior vena cava, and inferior vena cava.

- Veins all carry deoxygenated blood (except the pulmonary vein) from different body parts to the heart.

- Veins can be classified based on their positions. They can be superficial veins or deep veins.

- Connecting veins are short intermediary veins that connect the superficial and deep veins.

- Muscular compression and valves help to prevent a backflow of blood and propel blood towards the heart.

- Arteries generally transport oxygenated blood from the heart to the tissues, except for the pulmonary artery. The pulmonary artery transports deoxygenated blood (blood with low oxygen content) from the heart to the lungs.

- Arteries have a wall that comprises 3 major layers:
  - Tunica intima, which is the endothelium or inner layer.
  - Tunica media: Refers to the smooth muscle present in the arteries and expands or contracts as needed.
  - Tunica externa is the outer layer, and it communicates with other tissues and structures.

- The veins that are preferred, in order of choice, include the following:
  - Median cubital vein
  - Cephalic vein
  - Basilic vein
  - Dorsal venous network
  - Foot

CHAPTER THREE: THE BLOOD

"Blood is a very special juice." - Johann Wolfgang von Goethe

Blood is a tissue that is composed predominantly of water. Every adult has approximately 5.5 liters of blood. Blood is composed of two parts:

- The formed elements

- Plasma

Plasma

Plasma is the fluid within which the formed elements are suspended, and it forms about 55% of the blood in circulation. It is composed of water, proteins, electrolytes, hormones, sugars, amino acids, and waste products such as urea which are being transported for excretion.

Formed Elements

The formed elements refer to the cellular components of the blood, which represent 45% of the blood. The cells that are present in the blood include:

- Erythrocytes

- Leucocytes

- Thrombocytes

Erythrocytes

Erythrocytes are red blood cells. They get their red color from the iron-containing protein, hemoglobin, which is important in the transportation of oxygen. Erythrocytes are ellipsoid in shape, malleable, and typically have a normal lifespan of 120 days. There are usually about 4.2 to 6.2 million red blood cells (RBCs) present in one microliter of blood. RBCs are chiefly responsible for transporting oxygen to other cells and tissues in the body. They are also involved in the excretion and removal of CO_2 from the tissues, where they are generated to the lungs, where they are excreted. RBCs contain hemoglobin which is a good blood buffer. Red blood cells also carry antigens, such as the ABO and rhesus factor, which are important in blood transfusion and pregnancy.

Leucocytes

Leukocytes are white blood cells (WBCs), and they are the cells that defend the body against unwanted hosts and attacks. There are several types of leukocytes which include:

Neutrophils: The most prevalent type of leucocyte, forming between 40 and 70% of the total leucocyte population. They have fine granules present in their cytoplasm. They attack bacteria by phagocytosis; that is, they ingest the bacteria to eliminate the threat. They are usually the first responders when there is an infection.

Lymphocytes: are the second most prevalent type of leukocytes. They typically have a bean-shaped nucleus and lack granules in their cytoplasm. They form between 20 and 40% of the total WBC count in the body, and they are divided into two classes:

- T-lymphocytes involved in cellular immunity.

- B-Lymphocytes, which are responsible for humoral immunity.

Monocytes: are the largest type of WBCs. They also lack granules in their cytoplasm and have a nucleus that is either central or pushed to one corner of the cell. Once they get into tissues, they become macrophages which are involved in phagocytosis. They represent about 3 -8% of the total WBC count in the body.

Eosinophils: These are involved in attacking foreign bodies that antibody molecules have labeled. They are also implicated in allergies and skin reactions. They form about 1 - 3% of the body's total WBC count.

Basophils: These are WBCs with a bilobed nucleus. They are involved in allergic reactions in which they release histamine. They form about 0 - 1% of the WBC population.

The total WBC count is usually between 4000 - 11000/cubic millimeters of blood.

Thrombocytes/Platelets

These are known as thrombocytes or platelets. They are minute, anucleated bodies that are formed in the bone marrow. They are adhesive, aggregate easily, and agglutinate (clump together). These features are very important to the functions that they perform. These include blood clotting, clot retraction, and hemostasis (preventing excessive loss of blood). They are usually between 140000-400000 per microliter of blood and typically live for about 9 - 12 days.

The Immune System

Immunity refers to the ability of the body to fight infections. When foreign bodies like bacteria, viruses, and fungi invade the body, immunity enables the body to fight back. Immunity is broadly classified into two categories:

1. Innate immunity

2. Acquired immunity

Innate immunity refers to the inborn ability of the body to resist infectious agents. It is usually the first line of defense of the body against different pathogens. Innate immunity is also referred to as non-specific immunity because the response is the same regardless of the kind of pathogen or agent that attacks the body.

Some of the mechanisms of innate immunity include:

- Barriers: both anatomical and physiological.

- Activation of the complement system, which facilitates the destruction of invading microorganisms.

- Secretion of cytokines.

- Presence of enzymes in digestive juices in the gastrointestinal tract, which destroys harmful substances.

- Phagocytosis exhibited by neutrophils and macrophages.

Acquired immunity, also known as specific immunity, is resistance the body develops against specific pathogens or foreign bodies. It is more powerful but usually slower than non-specific or innate immunity. The lymphocytes mediate both types of immunity.

Acquired immunity can be divided into:

- Cellular immunity

- Humoral immunity

Cellular immunity is the function of T lymphocytes (T Cells) which are processed in the thymus. Cell-mediated immunity is the type of immune response that the body produces without antibodies. Instead, macrophage activation and NK-cells (Natural Killer cells) are produced. This type of immunity is very efficient in destroying cells that are infected with viruses, bacteria, or even cancers.

Humoral immunity is a function of the B Lymphocytes (B Cells), which are processed in the liver in utero and in the bone marrow after birth. The production of antibodies characterizes humoral immunity in response to the presence of an antigen on the surface of a pathogenic cell. This antigen binds to a specific receptor on the B Cell, which then stimulates a response that then stimulates the production of numerous plasma cells, which then secrete large quantities of antibody molecules. Antibodies circulating in the blood can bind to microorganisms like viruses and bacteria and interfere with their chemical reactions. They can also prevent them from entering other cells of the host. Antibodies can also mark pathogenic cells in opsonization so that phagocytic cells (e.g., neutrophils, macrophages) can locate and destroy them.

Hemostasis

Hemostasis simply refers to the stoppage of bleeding. The series of steps results in the cessation of bleeding from blood vessels.

Hemostasis occurs in the following stages:

- **Vasoconstriction:** This happens immediately after the injury to the blood vessel. The injury to the blood vessel endothelium causes collagen to be exposed. The affected blood vessel constricts to reduce its lumen and blood flow from the damaged portion. It is important to understand that this vasoconstriction is not systemic. It is local to where the injury has occurred and is usually limited to the arterioles and small arteries. Serotonin, secreted by the platelets, and other substances also add to the vasoconstriction at this stage. Here also, the platelets exhibit adherence to the exposed collagen, facilitated by a factor known as the Von Willebrand factor.

- **Formation of the platelet plug:** The platelet plug is formed from the platelets. After adherence of platelets to the exposed collagen of the damaged blood vessel, they begin to secrete ADP and Thromboxane A2. These two substances then attract even more platelets. All these platelets aggregate to form a platelet plug, which is temporary and seabed to close up the damaged blood vessel and prevent excessive blood loss.

- **Blood coagulation:** In this process, the conversion of fibrinogen to fibrin takes place and completely blocks the damaged blood vessel and prevents blood loss permanently. Converting fibrinogen to fibrin requires several coagulation factors and a coagulation cascade.

This cascade has three stages:

1. The formation of the prothrombin activator occurs via 2 pathways which are the intrinsic and extrinsic pathways.

2. The conversion of prothrombin into thrombin.

3. The conversion of fibrinogen to fibrin.

After clot formation, fibrinolysis is the breakdown and removal of the clot from inside the blood vessel.

In monitoring the coagulation cascades, some tests are used.

These are:

- APTT (Activated Partial Thromboplastin Time): Used to monitor the intrinsic pathway.

- Prothrombin time (PT): Used in the evaluation of the extrinsic pathway.

CHAPTER SUMMARY

- The blood is composed of two portions: the formed elements and plasma.

- Plasma is the fluid within which the formed elements are suspended, and it forms about 55% of the blood in circulation.

- The formed elements refer to the cellular components of the blood, which represent 45% of the blood.

The cells that are present in the blood include:

- Erythrocytes
- Leucocytes
- Thrombocytes

- Erythrocytes are red blood cells. They get their red color from the iron-containing protein, hemoglobin, which is important in the transportation of oxygen.

- Leukocytes are white blood cells, and they are the cells that defend the body against unwanted hosts and attacks.

There are several types of leukocytes which include:

- Neutrophils: The most prevalent type of leucocyte. They are usually the first responders when there is an infection.

- Lymphocytes: are the second most prevalent type of leukocytes.

They are divided into two classes:

  - T-lymphocytes involved in cellular immunity.

  - B-Lymphocytes, which are responsible for humoral immunity.

- Monocytes: are the largest type of white blood cells. Once they get into tissues, they become macrophages which are involved in phagocytosis.

- Eosinophils: are involved in attacking foreign bodies that antibody molecules have labeled. They are also implicated in allergies and skin reactions.

- Basophils: are WBCs with a bilobed nucleus. They are involved in allergic reactions in which they release histamine.

- Platelets are also known as thrombocytes. Their functions include blood clotting, clot retraction, and hemostasis (preventing excessive loss of blood).

- Immunity refers to the ability of the body to fight infections. Immunity is broadly classified into two categories:
    - Innate immunity

- Acquired immunity

- Innate immunity refers to the inborn ability of the body to resist infectious agents.

- Acquired immunity, also known as specific immunity, is resistance the body develops against specific pathogens or foreign bodies.

  Acquired immunity can be divided into:
  - Cellular immunity (Mediated by T cells)
  - Humoral immunity (Mediated by B Cells)

- Hemostasis simply refers to the stoppage of bleeding.
- It occurs in the following stages: vasoconstriction, formation of platelet plug, blood coagulation.

In monitoring the coagulation cascades, some tests are used. These are:

- Activated Partial Thromboplastin Time (APTT) is used to monitor the intrinsic pathway.

- Prothrombin time (PT) is used to evaluate the extrinsic pathway.

CHAPTER FOUR: PHLEBOTOMY PROCEDURES – VENIPUNCTURE

"Phlebotomists: We are vein people." - Unknown

The major phlebotomy procedure is venipuncture. Some people equate venipuncture to phlebotomy, but that is not correct. Phlebotomy as a field is more than venipuncture. It also involves other sample collection forms, such as fingerstick sampling and arterial blood collection. It also involves the care of samples collected, the labeling, and other things involved.

Venipuncture is just the process of collecting the sample from a vein. It is the most common way of sample collection in phlebotomy.

Patient identification and preparation

- Before carrying out any sample collection, the first thing to do is to prepare the patent and materials for the procedure.

- Ensure that there is a requisition form for every patient. This form must contain the following information:

  - Patient's name in full

  - Patient's hospital ID number

  - Government-issued ID cards can also be useful for the identification of patients.

- The date of birth and sex of the patient.

- The full name of the requesting physician.

- The sample to be collected, that is, blood.

- The test for which the sample is meant, for instance, full blood count, electrolytes urea, and creatinine.

- Ask for any allergies or patient sensitivities to antiseptics or latex, which are part of the materials to be used.

- If a patient is not conscious or unable to respond, then a phlebotomist should check the armband or bracelet or ask the nursing staff or relations for the patient's full name.

If the patient is conscious, explain what you want to do and why you need to do it so they can be mentally prepared. This is important because some patients, especially those who have been admitted to hospital for a long duration, would have taken so many samples from them and might be wondering why another sample is necessary or why you must prick them again. Speaking to them would also reassure them about the process.

Factors to consider before performing a venipuncture.

After going through the order, the following factors should be considered based on the information provided.

1. **Fasting:** Some tests require a patient to attend the phlebotomist fasting, such as fasting blood sugar (FBS). The phlebotomist should confirm this and ensure that

the patient has not had any food in the last 12 hours. This is very important, as eating before a test that should be done fasting would greatly alter the test results. If the patient has eaten, the test has to be postponed to another day when they are fasting.

2. **Edema:** When there is edema, in the upper limb especially, there is a high possibility of incorrect results. Therefore, the contralateral limb should be used in patients who have done a mastectomy on one side.

3. **Fistulas:** are arteriovenous connections and should be avoided in venipuncture as they can lead to infection.

4. **Timing:** Some tests are better done in the morning when their levels in the blood are optimal so that an accurate result can be obtained of the function of the substance. A good example of this is cortisol. The timing factor is closely related to the fasting factor because there is a higher chance that a patient has not had anything overnight when they come in the morning.

5. **Urgency of the test**: Some tests must be carried out urgently, and a phlebotomist must act accordingly. A very good example is in a case of mass casualties or emergencies, when a patient is bleeding, and the PCV or full blood count is needed to make an immediate decision. Speed and accuracy are extra important at this point, as the samples need to be taken in time.

6. **Age of the patient:** Adults can usually cooperate willingly when phlebotomists who want to take samples. With children however, phlebotomists might need assistance from their parents and other healthcare staff to steady the child and not disrupt the procedure.

Materials needed for the procedure

1. **Antiseptic:** Most common antiseptic that is used is 70% isopropyl alcohol. Povidone iodine is used for swabs if the sample to be taken is for blood culture. Chlorhexidine gluconate is another excellent option in place of povidone iodine.

2. **Tourniquet:** The tourniquet is used to stop the flow of blood through the veins to the heart. When this happens, the vein bulges from the point of the tourniquet backward, and this helps to locate the veins easily. There are different types, but the latex strip is the most common.

3. **Vacutainer needles:** These come in different sizes, but the 1.0-inch and 1.5-inch needles are commonly used. They are single use.

4. **Sterile syringes and needles:** These can also be used when vacutainer needles are not available. They cannot be reused.

5. **Butterfly winged infusion sets:** Useful in pediatric or elderly patients or small veins.

6. **Gloves:** Should be worn at all times by the phlebotomist before taking the sample. They protect the phlebotomist from infection and prevent contamination of the sample.

7. **Specimen bottles:** Specimen bottles should be available before the commencement of the procedure. These bottles should be appropriately labeled with the patient's name and identification number.

8. **Good source of light:** Sample collection should never be attempted where the lighting is not bright enough.

PROCEDURE

- Ensure the requisition is valid and verified.

- Patient identification and preparation are all done (including fasting if necessary, timing, etc., as previously discussed).

- Introduce yourself and explain the procedure to be done.

- Palpation of the veins in the elbow region with your index finger, mark the notable vein you will use.

- Gather all the necessary equipment that would be needed.

- Wash your hands and wear your gloves.

- Apply the tourniquet. The tourniquet should be applied to about 3 to 4 inches above the site you have selected for the venipuncture.

- The patient should make a fist, not pump the hand.

- Palpate the vein and feel for the point straight enough for the needle.

- Clean the site with alcohol in a circular motion starting from the intended position of venipuncture and outward.

- Uncap the needle and allow the site to dry.

- Hold the patient's arm below the site to tighten the skin and make the vein taut.

- Insert the needle with the bevel turned upwards at an angle of 15 to 30 degrees to the surface of the arm. The insertion should be swift and precise into the vein's lumen. Do not probe excessively.

- Once the last tube to be drawn is filled, loosen the tourniquet. Once blood flow has been established, the tourniquet should not be kept in place for more than two minutes. However, for the NHA examination, removing the tourniquet after one minute or once blood flow has been established is the correct thing to do. This is in order to prevent hemoconcentration of the samples collected.

- Samples should be taken in what is called the 'order of draw.'

Order of Draw

The correct order of draw as stated by the NHA is:

1. Blood culture bottles or vials

2. Sodium citrate bottles - (blue cover)

3. Serum tubes or plain bottles (without clot activator) – (red cover)

4. Heparin bottles – (green cover)

5. EDTA bottles - (lavender cover)

6. Oxalate/fluoride bottles - (gray cover)

- Once the bottles have been filled, withdraw the needle in a swift motion.

- Place a sterile gauze over the site and apply pressure to prevent the formation of a hematoma. (Asking the patient to bend the arm is not effective as this action does not provide enough pressure.)

- Discard the used needle and syringes into the biohazard sharps container.

- Label each specimen that has been collected. Include the name and hospital ID of the patient, the time and date sample was collected, and your name/initials.

- Now place the tubes inside the designated biohazards transport bag.

- Always check the venipuncture site before leaving the patient's side. If the bleeding has not stopped, apply more pressure for another two minutes. If it is still bleeding, apply for another 3 minutes. However, if bleeding does not stop after 8 minutes of pressure application, then the phlebotomist should call for help.

- Once the bleeding stops, an adhesive bandage should be placed over a sterile gauze.

- The place used for the procedure should be cleaned up, and all waste should be properly disposed of.

- Gloves should be removed and disposed of. Wash your hands.

- Thank the patient for their cooperation and inform them that their doctor will deliver the results.

Things to avoid

Take note of the following things to avoid before, during, and after the procedure:

- Labeling tubes before the procedure.

- Leaving the patient's side without labeling the tubes.

- Dismissing an outpatient when the tubes have not been labeled.

- Labeling specimen bottles with a pencil.

- Leaving the patient without ensuring that the bleeding from the venipuncture site has stopped.

Types of Bottles/Tubes Used in Sample Collection

- **Lavender top bottle/tube:** This is typically used in the collection of complete blood counts (CBC), ESR, blood group and hematocrit. It contains ethylenediaminetetraacetic acid (EDTA), which prevents blood clotting. It does this by binding calcium present in the blood sample. During collection, sample bottles/tubes should be about 2/3 full and inverted 8 times.

- **Red top bottle/tube:** This sample bottle is also known as the plain bottle because it contains no anticoagulants or additives. Here, blood clots normally on its own, after about thirty minutes of sample collection. It is used for serology tests and serum chemistry tests.

- **Light blue bottle/tube:** This sample bottle is used in coagulation studies, e.g., APTT (Activated Partial Thromboplastin Time), PT (Prothrombin Time), heparin therapy. It can do this because of the presence of sodium citrate. Sodium citrate is an anticoagulant which exerts its effect by binding to calcium. It is preferred for coagulation studies because it does not interfere with any of the coagulation factors. It should be filled and inverted about 3 to 4 times.

- **Green top bottle/tube:** Is also known as the heparin tube or bottle. It contains heparin, an anticoagulant mixed with either sodium, lithium or aluminum ions. Heparin inhibits the coagulation factor, thrombin. It is used in chemistry tests performed on plasma, e.g., ammonia. It is not routinely used in hematological tests because it interferes with one of the stains commonly used in hematology. (Wright's stain)

- **Gray top bottle/tube:** This sample bottle contains antiglycolytic agents, which aim to prevent the breakdown of glucose in the sample through different mechanisms. It usually contains sodium fluoride oxalate or lithium. Sodium fluoride and lithium both prevent the breakdown of glucose, while the oxalate present chelates calcium to prevent blood clotting. Samples should be inverted 8 times after collection. This bottle is typically used to collect fasting blood sugar, lactic acid, and glucose tolerance tests.

- **Yellow bottle/tube:** This sterile tube usually contains sodium polyanethol sulfonate (SPS). It is used in taking samples for culture. It should be inverted 8 times after sample collection.

Failure to obtain blood

In venipuncture, there can be several reasons for not obtaining blood. Some of the most common ones are:

- **Completely missing the vein:** The vein might be completely missed upon inserting the needle. To fix this, examine the position of the vein and the needle with a gloved finger and slowly redirect it.

- **Needle passed through the vein:** The needle is slowly withdrawn until it is fully back inside the vein to correct this. Usually, you would observe the flow of blood once the needle is fully in.

- **The needle is not fully inside the vein:** This would present as a flash of blood that would then stop flowing. Slowly push the needle into the vein so it enters fully.

- **Collapsed vein:** Sometimes the vein has collapsed, and blood does not flow out, no matter how the needle is adjusted. A collapsed vein might be because the vein has been used previously or the syringe or needle is too big for the vein. Here, the tourniquet should be removed, and another vein should be used for the sample collection.

- **Difficult vein:** Some veins are just difficult because of their positions. Some individuals have tiny or tortuous veins that make it difficult to get samples. Here, the phlebotomist has to be very careful and patient to prevent excessively pricking the patient. Smaller needles can be used if the arms are not.

- **Uncooperative patient:** Some patients might not be cooperative and/or might be shaky while taking the samples. This is especially true of pediatric patients and some adults with very low pain thresholds. The phlebotomist might need the assistance of relatives or other healthcare workers in these cases. Also, patients that have been in the hospital for a very long time might not be so cooperative if they have had venipuncture done many times. A phlebotomist must be very patient and reassuring to get them to cooperate. Samples should, as much as possible, be collected all at once and only when necessary to prevent inflicting unnecessary pain on the patient.

- **Fatigued personnel:** Sometimes, the phlebotomist has been working long hours and might be fatigued. Hence, they may not be able to get the vein for the required sample. Calling for help from other qualified health personnel to take the sample is always advisable instead of repeatedly pricking the patient. It also helps to avoid taking samples when the phlebotomists' concentration is low.

- **Poor peripheral circulation:** It might be very difficult to obtain samples from patients when there is poor peripheral circulation, as seen in the case of shock, severe bleeding or severe dehydration. When in shock, there is insufficient perfusion of tissues, and the body would shunt the rest of the blood to the most vital organs like the brain, and the peripheral circulation might suffer. In this kind of setting, samples might have to be taken via other methods such as the femoral tap.

Special Phlebotomy Procedures

The procedure described above is for routine venipuncture, which covers most phlebotomy procedures. However, some venipuncture procedures are carried out under special circumstances. They are regarded as "special", because of the requirement of timing, fasting, and other specific factors. Some of them include the following:

1. **Fasting specimens**

   Here, the patient must not eat for at least 12 hours before the specimen is taken. A good example is fasting blood glucose, which tests the blood sugar level without eating. Therefore, a phlebotomist must confirm that a patient has not eaten before the test is carried out.

2. **Timed specimens**

   These specimens are taken at specific times or in specific time sequences to obtain a specific result. They are usually used to evaluate the blood levels of substances that vary over time, for instance, cortisol, which exhibits diurnal variation. They are also used to determine the level of a substance or medication in the blood. A good example of this is digoxin. They are also used in the monitoring of a patient's condition. An example of this is a patient's hemoglobin level, which might have been observed to decrease over time. Also, after a blood transfusion, a PCV check might be required after 8 hours to see the new blood level.

3. **The Oral Glucose Tolerance Test (OGTT)** is one of the tests used to diagnose diabetes mellitus. It can be a 3hr OGTT or 5hr OGTT.

4. **Two-hour postprandial test**

This test is used to diagnose diabetes mellitus. The fasting blood sugar is compared against the blood sugar level 2 hours after a meal.

5. Blood cultures

Blood culture samples are taken to check for the presence and identity of microorganisms in the patient's blood. This is usually done when there is suspected septicemia. The test is usually carried out aseptically, with blood culture bottles. The test samples should be taken to the laboratory as soon as they are collected because the results are affected by temperature and the passage of time.

6. Phenylketonuria test

This test is carried out to screen for the presence of phenylalanine in the condition known as phenylketonuria. Phenylalanine buildup can affect the brains of children, cause developmental delays and intellectual disabilities. It is an inheritable disease and must be detected at birth to prevent complications. The sample used for this test is a few drops of blood taken from the newborn's heel.

7. Drug monitoring

Drug monitoring for therapeutic purposes is another specialized procedure in phlebotomy. Here samples are taken at timed sequences to monitor the concentration of the medication in the blood. The timing and frequency of the order for samples would depend on the drug's nature and the medication's purpose. Blood samples are taken to determine the lowest or trough level and peak level of concentration. Usually, trough-level samples are taken about 30 minutes before administering the first dose. Timing for the peak value would depend on the nature of the drug (half-life, clearance rate), the administration route, and the patient's metabolism rate.

Complications of Phlebotomy

As with any medical procedure, phlebotomy has several complications which a phlebotomist must know and avoid. It should be limited when it cannot be avoided, and the patient should be reassured.

1. **Formation of hematoma:** This is by far the most common complication of phlebotomy, especially during venipuncture. What happens is that blood flows out of the vein into the surrounding tissue. It usually occurs when the needle passes completely through the vein or when inadequate pressure is applied after the procedure. However, it is a temporary complication, and the hematoma should resolve within a few days after the procedure, although some can take longer. It is generally not a serious complication and should be resolved without intervention. Patients should, however, be advised to contact their doctor if they observe continuous swelling of the site, serious increasing discomfort, or numbness of the arm. It is best, however, to avoid this complication by ensuring that adequate pressure is applied to the venipuncture site after the procedure.

2. **Pain:** Almost any invasive procedure results in pain. The pain can be reduced by ensuring the phlebotomist gets a good vein that is visible enough to prevent excessive pricking.

3. **Hemoconcentration**: Refers to an increase in the ratio of formed elements of the blood to the plasma volume. It is usually caused by leaving the tourniquet on the patient for an extended period (greater than 2 minutes). It can lead to incorrect

or altered results. It can be avoided by removing the tourniquet once blood flow is established.

4. **Trauma:** Trauma happens to the underlying tissues when there is excessive probing with the needle during the procedure. Trauma to the skin is also inevitable as the needle has to enter through the skin to access the vein. It can be, however, reduced by limiting the extent of probing during sample collection. The phlebotomist should ensure they have a good, visible vein from which blood can be taken with minimal probing and injury to the client.

5. **Phlebitis:** This means there is inflammation of a vein. Phlebitis usually results from multiple venipunctures in a particular vein. Repeating venipuncture on the same vein should be avoided as much as possible. Apart from the inflammation, it can also be very painful to the patient.

6. **Thrombus formation and thrombophlebitis:** Thrombus (blood clot) formation can happen when inadequate pressure is applied on the venipuncture site after the needle is withdrawn. Thrombophlebitis means blood clot formation along with inflammation of the vein. Both can be avoided by applying adequate pressure after the procedure.

7. **Petechiae:** These refer to tiny, flat red spots that appear on the skin after the procedure. They are caused by capillary ruptures that can result from the tourniquet being left on for too long.

8. **Septicemia:** This occurs when microorganisms are introduced into the body via venipuncture. This can be avoided by following all aseptic procedures seriously and ensuring the sterility of all materials introduced into the patient's body.

9. **Extensive injuries/wounds:** Blood samples from certain patients at the wrong sites can lead to extensive injury. For instance, when samples are taken from the foot in diabetic patients, it can result in diabetic foot disease if the site refuses to close up and is improperly managed.

10. **Excessive bleeding:** Certain patients might have conditions where bleeding does not stop in time and can be excessive. Bleeding can also result if the needle is pushed into an artery. The phlebotomist should call for help if blood flow does not stop after 8 minutes.

11. **Needle prick (self-injury):** During the procedure, a phlebotomist can get injured while trying to take samples. This can result in infection or transmission of certain diseases, for instance hepatitis B or HIV, from the patient. To avoid this, needles should never be recapped once they are used. Needles should be safely disposed into the designated sharps box. Samples should only be taken when there is a good source of light. Samples should not be taken when the patient is uncooperative without assistance, especially in pediatric patients and infants.

CHAPTER SUMMARY

- Venipuncture is simply the process of collecting the sample from a vein. It is the most common type of sample collection in phlebotomy.

- Before carrying out any sample collection, the first thing to do is to prepare the patient and materials for the procedure.

- Factors to consider before performing a venipuncture include fasting, edema, fistulas, timing, urgency of the test, and age of the patient.

- Materials such as antiseptic, tourniquets, vacutainer needles, sterile syringes, etc. should be assembled before starting the procedure.

- The correct order of draw as stated by the NHA is:
  - Blood culture bottles or vials
  - Sodium citrate bottles (blue cover)
  - Serum tubes or plain bottles (without clot activator) (red cover)
  - Heparin bottles (green cover)
  - EDTA bottles (lavender cover)
  - Oxalate/fluoride bottles (gray cover)

- The lavender top bottle/tube: This is typically used in the collection of complete blood counts (CBC), ESR, blood group and hematocrit. It contains ethylenediaminetetraacetic acid (EDTA), which prevents blood clotting.

- Red top bottle/tube: This sample bottle is also known as the plain bottle because it contains no anticoagulants or additives. It is used for serology tests and serum chemistry tests.

- Light blue bottle/tube: This sample bottle is used in coagulation studies, e.g., APTT (Activated Partial Thromboplastin Time), PT (Prothrombin Time), heparin therapy. It can do this because of the presence of sodium citrate.

- Green top bottle/tube: It contains heparin, an anticoagulant mixed with either sodium, lithium or aluminum ions. It is used in chemistry tests performed on plasma, e.g., ammonia.

- Gray top bottle/tube: Contains antiglycolytic agents, which aim to prevent the breakdown of glucose in the sample through different mechanisms. This bottle is typically used to collect fasting blood sugar, lactic acid, and glucose tolerance tests.

- This sterile tube usually contains sodium polyanethol sulfonate (SPS). It is used for taking samples for culture.

- Special phlebotomy procedures include fasting specimens, timed specimens, OGTT, 2hr post prandial, blood cultures, PKU test, and drug monitoring.

- Complications of phlebotomy include formation of hematoma, pain, hemoconcentration, trauma, phlebitis, thrombophlebitis, petechiae, septicemia, extensive injuries/wounds, etc.

GET YOUR FREE BONUSES

Dear reader,

First and foremost, thank you for purchasing my book! Your support means the world to me, and I hope you find the information within valuable and helpful in your phlebotomy journey.

As a token of my appreciation, I have included some exclusive bonuses that will greatly benefit you in your career.

Your Bonuses:

1. **The Phlebotomy Success Blueprint**: This exclusive ebook is your secret weapon to outsmart the competition and stand out in the highly competitive phlebotomy industry. With this blueprint, you'll unlock your earning potential, discover amazing career opportunities, and get insider tips that will set you apart from the rest.

2. **100 Phlebotomy Flashcards**: These digital and printable flashcards are an excellent tool to help you study and retain crucial phlebotomy information. They are designed to reinforce your knowledge, boost your confidence, and make learning enjoyable and convenient, whether you're on-the-go or at home.

3. **Complete Quick-Reference Phlebotomy Guide**: This handy guide covers the most important topics and techniques in phlebotomy, making it an invaluable resource for last-minute studying and quick reference during your daily work. Its concise and easy-to-understand format will save you time and help you feel well-prepared for any situation.

I kindly ask you to take a moment to leave an honest review of the book. Your feedback not only helps me improve my future work, but it also assists other readers in making informed decisions on their purchases. Please share your thoughts and experiences, as every review counts!

To access these bonuses, simply click on the link if you're using the ebook version, or scan the QR Code with your phone if you have the physical copy.

CLICK   HERE   FOR   THE   BONUSES

or
Scan this QR Code

Once again, thank you for your support, and I wish you the best of luck in your phlebotomy career. I believe these bonuses will provide you with the tools and knowledge to excel in this industry.

If you want to leave an honest review, here's the link for direct access:

Or, Scan this QR Code below

Happy reading, and enjoy your bonuses!

CHAPTER FIVE: PHLEBOTOMY PROCEDURES - DERMAL PUNCTURE

"Phlebotomy is a bloody job, but somebody's got to do it." - Anonymous

A dermal puncture is a phlebotomy procedure performed when venipuncture might not be possible or when just a little sample of blood is required. Therefore, it is unsuitable for tests requiring a larger amount of blood or serum, e.g., blood cultures or ESR.

Dermal punctures should be performed with a lancet, usually with predetermined depth values (0.85mm recommended for infants, 3.0mm recommended for adults). Avoid using hypodermic needles or surgical blades for dermal punctures because the incision might be difficult to control and can result in excessive bleeding and injury. It can also introduce infection into the body.

Sites for Dermal Puncture

In infants, the preferred site for punctures is the heel (plantar surface of the foot), at the medial and lateral regions. According to the American Academy of Pediatrics (AAP), heel punctures should not exceed a depth of 2.0mm in infants. Also, the puncture should not be performed on sites that have been used previously, and the appropriate sites should be used for the procedure.

The distal portion of the 3rd or 4th finger is typically used in older children and adults. The non-dominant hand of the patient should be used for this procedure. The puncture should be made in a direction perpendicular to the fingerprint lines.

Procedure

- Patient identification, as stated for the venipuncture.

- Preparation and assembly of materials.

- The site should be prewarmed using a towel that has been moistened with warm water for about 3 minutes. Warming the site before puncture helps to greatly increase the flow of blood to the finger.

- Handwashing and wearing of gloves.

- Clean the site with 70% isopropyl alcohol and allow it to dry. Avoid povidone-iodine for this procedure as it interferes with several results.

- Use the puncture device to perform the puncture following the order of draw.

The order of draw for puncture specimens.

  - Lavender colored tubes.

  - Tubes with additives present.

  - Tubes with additives absent.

- Ensure that samples are properly labeled, using the same protocol as venipuncture.

- The patient should apply pressure with a sterile gauze to the puncture site once sample collection is over.

- Check the puncture site and ensure that the bleeding has stopped.

- Thank the patient and dispose of all materials appropriately.

- Remove gloves and wash hands.

- The sample should be placed in the biohazard specimen bag and delivered to the laboratory.

Limitations of Dermal Puncture

- It cannot be used to collect samples requiring a larger amount of blood, e.g., blood culture, ESR.

- Dermal puncture cannot be used if a patient is dehydrated.

- Dermal puncture cannot be used if a patient has a poor peripheral circulation.

- It can result in hemolysis or clot formation if there is a delay in the collection of blood samples, which can lead to rejection of samples at the laboratory or alteration of results.

- Air bubbles can enter the tube and prevent adequate samples from being taken.

CHAPTER SUMMARY

- A dermal puncture is a phlebotomy procedure performed when venipuncture might not be possible or when just a small sample of blood is required.

- In infants, the preferred site for punctures is the heel (plantar surface of the foot), at the medial and lateral regions.

- The distal portion of the 3rd or 4th finger is typically used in older children and adults.

- The order of draw for puncture specimens.

- Lavender colored tubes.
- Tubes with additives present.
- Tubes with additives absent.

- Dermal puncture cannot be used when a patient is dehydrated or has poor peripheral circulation. It is affected by delay in sample collection. Air bubbles can also enter the tube.

CHAPTER SIX: QUALITY ASSURANCE AND CONTROL

"Quality is never an accident. It is always the result of intelligent effort." – John Ruskin

Quality Assurance (QA) refers to systems, methods, and protocols that are set in place to ensure that a product or service meets the expected or specified requirements. Quality control becomes non-negotiable with systems that rely heavily on human involvement. This is because any system that has heavy human involvement has a higher chance of errors. Phlebotomy and healthcare, in general, are such fields.

In healthcare and more precisely, phlebotomy, QA must always be happening. This helps evaluate processes to reduce and eliminate errors, redundancy and improve the quality of healthcare delivery. It involves clearly stated guidelines for performing different services and continuous education of employees on findings and areas that should be improved.

Some areas that are continuously subjected to quality control include: patient preparation before collection, during the collection process and after collection. These errors, their solutions, and preventions will now be discussed in detail.

Before sample collection: These refer to errors that take place before the sample is collected. They include the misidentification of patients, wrong time of sample collection, usage of wrong tubes, inadequate fasting for samples that require fasting, wrong patient position, improper site selection and preparation, and/or interference of medication.

To avoid all these, all patients must be properly prepared before any phlebotomy procedure. Preparation begins with the state of the patient. For instance, are they fasting when they should be? Is the timing of the sample collection correct? The phlebotomist must ensure that all these are sorted even before beginning the collection of samples.

Patients should be asked to say their full names before starting any procedure. Patients should be rightly positioned for the procedure. If the patient is not conscious, a relative or nurse can help to position them well. The site for any phlebotomy procedure should be well prepared using the discussed protocols.

A phlebotomist should know about medications that might interfere with the samples being collected and ask the patient if they are taking any before they start the procedure.

During sample collection: Errors that occur during the collection of the sample include prolonged tourniquet time, hemolysis, blood clot formation, inappropriate order of draw, tube inversion done inadequately or not done at all, poor technique in sample collection, delays in taking the complete sample, and/or not taking enough sample for the test.

The phlebotomist must know what is required for each sample to avoid all these. The tourniquet should be removed once blood flow is established and avoid having it on for more than two minutes. Blood samples should be taken swiftly and with the appropriate needle sizes to prevent hemolysis. The right technique should be used for any phlebotomy procedure, and the sample tubes/bottles should be filled up to the specified mark. Most tubes usually have the specified mark on the labels.

After sample collection: Some of the common errors that happen here include inappropriate use of serum separator, failure of serum-cell separation, delays in sample processing, exposing some samples to light inappropriately, poor storage conditions, rimming clots from overexposure of sample to air and/or failure to invert immediately after collection.

To prevent some of these errors after sample collection, the phlebotomist must be vigilant and fast. You should always remember that irreversible changes begin to occur once the samples are taken out of the body. It, therefore, becomes a race against time between the phlebotomist and these changes that are rapidly occurring. The additives in the tubes or bottles can help slow down or reduce these changes, but the goal is to present these samples in a condition that is as close to the real in-vivo state of the patient as possible.

The samples must be collected using the right tubes. If not, the samples can't be used. Once samples are collected, they should be inverted the specified number of times, so that the additives can mix well with the sample and perform their functions.

The phlebotomist should also ensure that samples sensitive to light should be stored in dark containers or appropriate alternatives and stores. Exposure to air should be very limited, and there should be no delays in transporting the samples to the laboratory for processing. Some hospitals have staff that transport these samples. Ensure you follow up on these so that samples are not misplaced or lost in transit.

Handling of Special Specimen

Collected samples must be handled properly to ensure the quality of samples and the accuracy of results. Generally, the rules of ensuring fast transport, processing, and analysis should be followed for all samples. All samples should be properly accounted for, and proper records taken at every point, from collection to transportation, reception at the laboratory, analysis, and documentation of results. Part of the Quality Control after sample collection is ensuring that there are no errors in the results.

However, some samples have specific requirements:

1. Light-sensitive specimens: Some test results can be altered when the sample used for the test has been exposed to light. Examples of such tests include bilirubin tests, beta-carotene tests, and tests for porphyrins.

    To protect them, samples taken for these tests should be immediately wrapped with aluminum foil once they are drawn.

2. Cold specimens: Samples for tests such as arterial blood gasses, lactic acid, ammonia, ACTh, should all be placed inside containers with ice packs or crushed ice to keep them cold and immediately transported to the laboratory for processing.

3. Warm specimen: Some other samples require higher temperatures for storage and processing. An excellent example is the direct Coombs test, which requires that samples are placed in ordered containers at 37 - 38 degrees Celsius to remove serum or plasma.

Clinical Laboratory Sections

A phlebotomist should not just understand how to take blood samples. Phlebotomists should have at least a basic understanding of where the samples go when they are taken to the laboratory.

Generally, hospital laboratories consist of about 6 sections:

- Hematology section

- Chemistry section

- Blood bank

- Serology/Immunology section

- Microbiology

- Urinalysis

Each of these sections can be further subdivided into smaller units. However, most laboratories have these sections to handle the day-to-day tests of the hospital.

Hematology section

At the hematology section, blood, and its elements, both formed and fluid are studied. The tests that are usually carried out here include:

Complete blood count: This separates the formed elements of the blood into the red blood cells, white blood cells, neutrophils, lymphocytes, monocytes, basophils, eosinophils and platelets. It also shows the hematocrit, mean corpuscular volume and mean corpuscular hemoglobin concentration (MCHC).

Erythrocyte Sedimentation Rate (ESR): The ESR is a measure of the inflammatory activity going on in the body. It measures the rate of sedimentation of RBCs, that is, the rate at which Red Blood cells fall to the bottom of a Westergren tube. Generally, when there is inflammation, RBCs would fall faster, thus having a higher sedimentation rate, and consequently elevated ESR.

Coagulation studies: These also take place in the hematology sections in some laboratories. In other labs, they have their own section. However, the tests that commonly take place in the coagulation section are:

APTT (Activated Partial Thromboplastin Time): This is used to test for all the factors involved in the intrinsic and common pathways. It does this by measuring the time it takes that particular sample to form a cot after exposure to calcium and a phospholipid emulsion. The normal reference range is 30 -40 seconds.

TT (Thrombin Time): Refers to the time spent for fibrinogen to be converted to fibrin. Thrombin is the catalyst of that step, so when thrombin is added to the sample, the time it takes to bring about this effect is known as Thrombin time.

PT (Prothrombin Time): This test measures the time it takes for blood to clot via the extrinsic pathway. Therefore, it measures the efficiency of the irrelevant and the common pathways. This test requires the tube to be about 60-80% full because of the presence of citrate, a common anticoagulant used in the sample collection. Adequate blood creates a high blood volume to anticoagulant volume ratio. Usually, the INR (International Normalized Ratio) is derived from the PT and used to calculate a more widely accepted value independent of the variations caused by the reagent used.

Other tests in the hematology section include bleeding time, reticulocyte count, peripheral blood film sickle cell, etc.

Chemistry Section

In the chemistry section, analysis of body fluids takes place using biochemical reactions. These reactions are used to identify and quantify the different components present in body fluids. The chemistry section also uses a lot of automation to analyze samples and generate results.

The most common specimens that are tested in this section include blood, serum, plasma, urine and cerebrospinal fluid (CSF).

Tests that are carried out in this section include:

Electrophoresis: An electric field separates the blood into its chemical parts. The protein charge and structure differences eventually determine how far they can travel in this field. This principle is used to analyze blood components like hemoglobin. Electrophoresis is commonly used to determine the hemoglobin types in patients. It can also be used in serum, CSF, and urine.

Toxicology: Toxicology screening is very important in health facilities, as it can help rapidly detect the presence or absence of specific classes of drugs or poisons in a person's body. Toxicology screening would usually require blood or urine samples. They can also use saliva, hair, or sweat for the screening.

Immunochemistry: The science of studying the immune system and its responses. Immunohistochemistry makes use of the immune responses to identify and quantify different components in the body, such as antigens, hormones, enzymes, etc.

Other tests in this section usually combine several parameters into one profile of tests. For instance, the liver profile test is composed of alkaline phosphatase (ALP), alanine transaminase (ALT), aspartate transaminase (AST), gamma glutamyl transferase (GGT) and bilirubin (Direct and Total). All these tests have been developed to assess liver function and would provide results about different aspects of liver function.

Blood Bank

The blood bank is the section of the lab where the blood collection, preparation, and storage are done for transfusion. There are very strict protocols here for identifying patients and handling the specimen. Blood that is donated and collected here can be separated and packaged as whole blood, packed cells, fresh frozen plasma, platelets, or cryoprecipitate.

Usually, before donation happens, the donor is screened for common infections like hepatitis B and C, HIV/AIDS, and others. Their hematocrit level is checked to ensure it is not below the minimum for age and sex. Only after this, is blood donated, packaged and stored.

Serology/Immunology

Serology refers to the study of the body's serum, while immunology is defined as the study of the immune system. This laboratory section focuses on detecting antibodies to certain viruses, bacteria, fungi and other microorganisms. These antibodies are then used to determine the presence or absence, activity level, quantity, and type of microorganism that is present. For instance, the hepatitis B antibody, antibodies to HIV, etc.

Serology also helps to investigate disease conditions. This section involves autoimmune disorders, which happen when the body produces antibodies against its organs and tissues, and immunodeficiency disorders, which weaken the immune system. Usually, these antibodies that are produced can be used to closely monitor the progression of the disease.

Organ and tissue compatibility: This section also investigates the chances of acceptance or rejection of a body part in the case of a transplant.

Microbiology

The microbiology section is involved with identifying and quantifying parasites, pathogens, and microorganisms in the specimen provided. It is heavily involved in hospital infection control. Usually, the most common test is culture and sensitivity, which shows the type of organism and the drugs or antibiotics it is sensitive to. This is vital to prevent the abuse of antibiotics and to stop the infection quickly. These tests are also very useful when a patient is experiencing sepsis or fever of unknown origin. Some cultures can take a longer time for results to be out. Specimens typically used here are blood, urine, and sputum.

The microbiologists also work with other healthcare team members to determine the best protocols to contain and prevent infection, especially for hospital-acquired infection. They can inform or educate on good aseptic techniques and how to prevent contamination of samples.

Urinalysis Section

This section deals with everything related to urine, using the condition of urine to detect diseases, disorders, or infections that are present in the body. Some of the examinations that are carried out on the urine include:

Macroscopic examination: Is the process which looks at the physical properties of urine, such as the color, the smell clarity, and specific gravity.

Chemical examination: This deals with the chemical properties of urine, such as acidity, (pH) presence, and quantity of substances in the urine, such as glucose, ketones, proteins, blood, nitrites, WBCs.

Microscopic examination: This focuses on the presence of microscopic substances in the urine. For instance, the presence of casts and other microorganisms.

The tests that are performed on urine include:

Urinalysis: This is carried out with a strip containing chemical compounds that react with the chemical components in urine to test for their presence or absence.

The tests performed here also include urine microscopy, culture, and sensitivity, which detect the presence of bacteria, fungi and other pathogens in urine and the antibiotics they are sensitive to.

The information obtained from the urine can be especially useful in detecting disease conditions like diabetes mellitus, diabetes insipidus, urinary tract infection, along with their monitoring and their treatment.

CHAPTER SUMMARY

- Quality Assurance (QA) refers to systems, methods, and protocols that are set in place to ensure that a product or service meets the expected or specified requirements.

- Some areas that are continuously subjected to Quality Control include: patient preparation before collection, during the collection process and after collection.

- Errors before sample collection include misidentification of patients, wrong time of sample collection, usage of wrong tubes, inadequate fasting for samples that require fasting, wrong patient position, improper site selection and preparation, and/or interference of medication.

- Errors that occur during the collection of the sample include prolonged tourniquet time, hemolysis, blood clot formation, inappropriate order of draw, tube inversion done inadequately or not done at all, poor technique in sample collection, delays in taking the complete sample, not taking enough sample for the test.

- Errors that happen after collection include inappropriate use of serum separator, failure of serum-cell separation, delays in sample processing, exposing some samples to light inappropriately, poor storage conditions, rimming clots from overexposure of sample to air, failure to invert immediately after collection.

- Light-sensitive specimens: Some test results can be altered when the sample used for the test has been exposed to light. e.g., bilirubin tests. Samples taken for these tests should be immediately wrapped with aluminum foil once they are drawn.

- Cold specimens: Samples for tests such as arterial blood gasses, lactic acid, ammonia, ACTh, should all be placed inside containers with ice packs or crushed ices, to keep them cold and immediately transported to the laboratory for processing.

- Warm specimen: Some other samples require higher temperatures for storage and processing. An excellent example is the direct Coombs test.

- Generally, hospital laboratories consist of about 6 sections:

- Hematology section: Tests done here include CBC, ESR, coagulation studies.
- Chemistry section: Tests done here include electrophoresis, toxicology.
- Blood bank: Blood collection, preparation and storage are done for transfusion.
- Serology/Immunology section: HepB, and HIV tests are done here.
- Microbiology: Organ and tissue compatibility, as well as involved with identifying and quantifying parasites, pathogens, and microorganisms in the specimen provided.
- Urinalysis: This deals with using the condition of urine to detect diseases, disorders, or infections that are present in the body.

CHAPTER SEVEN: INFECTION CONTROL AND SAFETY

"Infection control is everybody's responsibility." – Sarah Green

Infection control and safety are critical components of any medical procedure. Phlebotomy, as a process that involves potential contact with blood and other bodily fluids, presents a high risk of transmitting infections from the patient to the healthcare provider and vice versa. Therefore, it is essential to follow proper infection control and safety procedures during phlebotomy to minimize the risk of transmission.

Infection control is not only important for ensuring the safety of the patient and attending phlebotomist but is also important for ensuring other healthcare providers, patients, and well-wishers who may interact with the patient of concern and equipment used do not become infected.

Therefore, infection control and safety measures" aim to ensure that everyone, including the patient of concern, the health workers, and other patients or individuals in healthcare settings, are at the least risk of contracting infection from phlebotomy procedures.

Overview of Infection Control

Infection control is a risk management approach that aims to ensure that infectious agents are not transmitted from one individual to another or, from one point to another during phlebotomy and other medical activities.

Microorganisms and infectious agents can be found everywhere. While most of them can be harmless, and some are even beneficial, there are also several microorganisms capable of compromising health and posing serious risks to whoever contracts them. Therefore, it is important that phlebotomist technicians understand how infection transmission works and how it can be curbed during their processes.

The Chain of Infection

Infection spreads through this definite chain:

Agent ------------> Mode of transmission ------------> Susceptible host

The link between the agent and the mode of transmission is the portal of exit, while the link between the mode of transmission and the susceptible host is the portal of entry.

Agents

Agents are the microorganisms responsible for causing infections. Agents are classified as viruses, bacteria, fungi, and parasites.

When medications are administered to treat infections, they are usually targeted toward the specific infection agent after it has been identified. This is why infection-treating medications exist in specific forms for treating bacterial, viral, and fungal infections.

Portal of Exit

The portal of exit is the passageway through which an infectious agent leaves its reservoir or initial host. Note that the portal of exit is not the medium that contains the agent but rather the route through which the medium, alongside the infectious agent, leaves a reservoir. Examples of portals of exit are the alimentary canal through actions such as coughing, vomiting, and diarrhea; the respiratory tract through actions such as sneezing; and the genitourinary tract through actions such as sexual intercourse, pregnancy, and childbirth.

Mode of Transmission

The mode of transmission is the specific way or medium that bears the infectious agent as it exits the reservoir. There are five important types of modes of transmission, which are:

· Contact (direct and indirect)

· Airborne

- Droplet

- Common vehicle

- Vector-borne

Portal of Entry

The portal of entry offers an entry point for the infectious agent into the susceptible host. Examples of portals of entry are broken skin, wound points, mucous membranes, and points where the respiratory, gastrointestinal, and urogenital tracts open to the external environment.

Susceptible Host

The susceptible host becomes the new host for the infectious agent after gaining access through the portal of entry. The success of an agent infecting the susceptible host would strongly depend on the immunity of the host as well as the resistance of the infection-causing agent. Once the susceptible host becomes infected, they become a reservoir through which the disease-causing agent can be transmitted to a new host.

Infection Control at Every Point in the Chain of Infection

Infection control is essential at every point in the chain of infection to limit the risk of transmission of infectious agents from one individual to the other. As already explained, the chain of infection involves six major points:

- The infectious agent

- The reservoir or initial host

- The portal of exit

- The mode of transmission

- The portal of entry

- The susceptible or new host

The Infectious Agent

Infection control at this point in the chain involves identifying the infectious agent, such as bacteria or viruses. While the phlebotomist technician may not be responsible for treating infection in patients, knowing exactly what infectious agents are present, if any, can guide the phlebotomist in utilizing the right precautionary measures.

Phlebotomists can retrieve information on a patient's infection state from their case files. In situations where blood is being collected for donation and transfusion processes, it is important that the donor is properly screened not only for blood compatibility but also for the presence of disease-causing infectious agents, even when they look healthy.

Donors might need to be treated for infection before donating or replaced altogether, to get viable blood. Retrieved blood may also go through sterilization and disinfection before they are transfused.

The Reservoir or Initial Host

Infection control, at this point, focuses on preventing the spread of infectious agents in the environment, such as contaminated surfaces or water. Measures can include proper sanitation, cleaning, and routine maintenance of the patient's environment. Equipment that is not single use should also be properly disinfected and sterilized before and after being used on a new patient.

The Portal of Exit

The portal of exit and portal of entry are important focus points for effective infection control since they are the only points in the phlebotomy process in which the phlebotomist technician has reasonable control and can ensure optimum protection.

The most relevant portal of exit to the phlebotomist is the bleeding site of the reservoir, but other exit points can also pose major risks. There are several standard precautions, transmission-based precautions, and protective equipment designed to prevent transmission of infection at this stage, whether for the patient or phlebotomist technician. The basic measures include wearing gloves, gowns, and masks, and covering coughs and sneezes.

Mode of Transmission

At this point, infection control is done by eliminating direct and indirect contact with any media that can transmit infection between the patient and the healthcare worker. These media include droplets, airborne particles, direct contact between the patient and care personnel, and indirect contact with already contaminated objects in the environment.

An important infection control method at this point is proper hand hygiene. Others include proper care of patients' environments, handling equipment properly, and the use of personal protective equipment that serves as barriers.

Portal of Entry

Like the portal of exit, the phlebotomist technician has adequate control of the portal of entry during the phlebotomy process. The phlebotomist must therefore play a crucial role in ensuring infectious agents do not pass into the patient.

Infection control and preventive measures at the portal of entry include transmission-based precautions during phlebotomy, sterile wound care, using the aseptic technique to minimize the transmission of infectious agents, and proper storage of collected blood and other bodily fluids.

Susceptible Host

As mentioned earlier, the success of the agent at infecting the susceptible host strongly depends on the immunity of the host and the resistance of the infection-causing agent to the immunity of the host.

Incurable diseases, for example, will be difficult to manage once they are transmitted into a new host. In whatever case, an important measure for curbing the further spread of infection is to separate the susceptible host from the reservoir and immediately begin to treat or manage the infection in the susceptible host.

An important precautionary measure before performing phlebotomy is to ensure that susceptible hosts are treated for underlying conditions that could compromise their immunity, while also ensuring that their immunity levels are at an optimal state.

Standard Precautions

Standard precautions in phlebotomy or any other healthcare practice are the precautions and routine activities that must be carried out in order to achieve a basic or minimal level of infection prevention and control. In other words, standard precautions are the minimum infection prevention and control practices that must be implemented when interacting with all patients, irrespective of what is known or not known about each patient.

Standard precautions are important because all living organisms and especially humans, potentially harbor infectious agents. These agents are transmitted through different media, of which blood and other body fluids are significant vehicles. Phlebotomists, who mostly interact with blood and other body fluids from patients, therefore, utilize these standard precautions to provide basic protection against infectious agents for the patient, themselves, and other persons actively in the healthcare environment.

Standard precautions in phlebotomy aim to reduce risk to the minimum level and, if possible, eliminate the risk altogether of transmitting bloodborne, disease-causing microorganisms.

Beyond standard precautions are the transmission-based precautions, which are used in situations where it has been determined that standard-based precautions will not suffice because the patient is suspected or has been diagnosed with a highly contagious disease-causing agent. More about transmission-based precautions will be discussed later on in this chapter.

Here are the standard precautions required of phlebotomy technicians:

Handwashing

Hand washing or hand hygiene is one of the basic yet most essential procedures for preventing and reducing the spread of infection. It is a routine practice that the phlebotomist technician must always pay attention to.

A simple routine hand washing procedure involves washing the hand with mild soap and running water. Certain hand washing procedures can, however, be more intense.

Hand antisepsis, for example, involves the use of antimicrobial soap when washing hands in order to kill or hinder the potency of microorganisms.

Hand rubbing, on the other hand, is the use of an alcohol-based hand rub (ABHR) for sanitizing the hand and hindering the potency of microorganisms. Hand rubbing is particularly used when the hand is not visibly soiled, or the hand is already clean as an additional layer of protection.

The World Health Organization (WHO) has recommended that hand hygiene should be done during the following five key moments:

· Before touching or coming in contact with a patient

· Before performing a procedure

· After performing a procedure (or after exposure to any bodily fluid from the patient)

· After touching the patient

· After touching the environment around the patient

Medical Asepsis

Medical asepsis is the procedure of destroying microorganisms and infectious agents after they've left the body. This ensures they are no longer potent to pose a risk to a patient or healthcare worker.

Medical asepsis involves procedures such as disinfection, equipment cleaning, and even hand washing after a phlebotomy procedure.

Medical asepsis can either be a standard precaution or a transmission-based precaution. It is standard procedure to always disinfect reusable equipment after completing a procedure. The knowledge of the situation and infection the phlebotomist is trying to curb can, however, guide the disinfection and equipment cleaning procedure to ensure the infection agent of concern is properly ridden off.

Note that disinfectants are used on medical equipment and not on human skin since they contain powerful chemicals that can irritate the skin and mucous membranes. Household bleach mixed with water in a ratio of 1:10 is a popular, non-expensive, and viable disinfectant that can be used for medical asepsis. Boiling water is also a viable disinfectant. It is, however, used only if the item to be disinfected will not be used in invasive procedures or other procedures where the equipment will be inserted into body orifices. Essentially, boiling water should not be used as the only disinfectant during procedures that require strict use of sterile equipment.

Medical asepsis is an extensive infection control process that extends to other activities, such as safe handling and properly disposing of sharp and contaminated materials. This will be discussed as a subsection of its own later on in this chapter.

Barrier Protection

As a standard precaution, phlebotomists and phlebotomist technicians should use protective clothing and other equipment to provide a barrier against infectious agents.

After using barrier protection, it is also important that they are disposed of properly, so they do not spread infections to others. To ensure this, it is important for the phlebotomist to understand the correct procedure for putting on and taking off each type of barrier protection, how to dispose of used equipment, and how to disinfect or sterilize reusable equipment for the next use.

Examples of barrier protection are gloves, masks, face shields, goggles, and respirators.

Isolation (of specimen)

isolation is an important standard precaution during phlebotomy and many other patient-care routines. The center for disease control (cdc) has recommended that all human blood and other bodily fluids should be considered potentially infectious and proper precautions should be taken to prevent the transmission of infections when interacting with these fluids.

The cdc recommends both standard and transmission-based precautions for isolation. As standard precautions for isolation, the cdc recommends that:

- o gloves should be worn when collecting and interacting with blood, other body fluids, or tissue specimens.
- o Face shields should be worn whenever there is a potential danger of splashing blood or body fluids on mucous membranes.
- o Needles and other sharp objects used should be disposed of in puncture-proof containers and left uncapped.

These are standard infection control practices that must be used with all patients during phlebotomy. These precautions are also generally used whenever there can be potential contact with some or all of the following:

- o blood
- o all kinds of body fluids, including secretions and excretions (excluding sweat), regardless of whether or not they contain visible blood
- o broken skin
- o mucous membranes
- o other recognized and unrecognized sources of infections

transmission-based precautions

transmission-based precautions are the infection prevention and control measures that are used when standard precautions alone will not suffice to prevent the spread of an infectious agent.

Transmission-based precautions are always specialized and tailored based on the type of infectious agent being prevented. This ensures that if the right measures are used, infection control is successful, and the safety of everyone will not be compromised. In situations when the suspected or diagnosed infectious agent has more than one mode of transmission, all the transmission-based precautions specific to that microorganism will be utilized.The three distinct categories of transmission-based precautions are:

- contact precautions
- airborne precautions
- droplet precautions

Isolation (of specimen)

specimen isolation procedures are used when the patient is suspected or has already been diagnosed as being infected with a contagious and disease-causing agent.

Contact precautions: contact precautions are designed to reduce the risk of transmission of infection-causing agents that can be transmitted by direct or indirect contact. Direct contact transmission refers to the transmission of infectious disease-causing agents through skin-to-skin contact or any other means that would directly transfer microorganisms from the reservoir to the susceptible host. Indirect contact transmission refers to the transmission of microorganisms that comes through contact with an intermediate object with which the reservoir patient has had contact.

Airborne precautions: airborne precautions are designed to reduce the risk of transmission of airborne infection-causing microorganisms. Such microorganisms and infectious agents are transported by air currents and can be easily contacted during activities like breathing and inhaling or when they come in direct contact with a vulnerable part of the susceptible host. Transmission-based airborne precautions typically include using ventilation and other special air handling techniques.

Droplet precautions: droplet precautions are designed to reduce the risk of infection-causing microorganisms transmitted by droplets. Infection through droplets usually occurs when there is contact with certain areas of the reservoir host, such as the mucous membranes of the nose or mouth, the conjunctivae, and during other activities such as sneezing, coughing, and talking. Droplet precautions do not typically include ventilation and other special air handling techniques since they do not travel far and do not remain suspended in the air for long.

Note that transmission-based precautions for isolation, as with all other transmission-based precautions, are to be used alongside standard isolation precautions. Transmission-based precautions do not overrule all other standard precautions that ought to be dutifully followed.

Personal protective equipment

personal protective equipment (ppe) is important for ensuring both standard and transmission-based infection precautions are maintained. Some ppe, such as those needed for standard precautions, must be readily available for the use of the phlebotomist technician every time. Other ppe for transmission-based precautions is utilized based on the nature of the infectious agent that is being prevented from spreading.

Gloves

gloves are worn as standard personal protective equipment to prevent the phlebotomists hands from exposure to blood and other body fluids. This in turn serves to protect three categories of people:

1.   The patient: by ensuring that infectious agents that have been on the hands of the healthcare personnel are not transmitted to the patient during procedures that require contact with the patient's risk areas for infection, such as broken skin and external openings of the gastrointestinal, respiratory, and urogenital tracts.

2.   The healthcare personnel: by ensuring that infectious agents are not transmitted from the patient to the healthcare worker during contact with broken skin, body fluids, secretions, and other transmission media of the patient.

3.   Other patients: by ensuring that infectious agents that may have contaminated the healthcare personnel are not transmitted to another patient. This is also the reason why gloves are single-use and are not shared between patients.

There are two distinct types of gloves: single-use or non-sterile gloves and sterile gloves. Sterile gloves are used during invasive procedures that require strict use of sterile equipment. Otherwise, single-use, non-sterile gloves would suffice for most phlebotomy procedures.

Note that although gloves are a standard precaution, they should not be used as an alternative or replacement for hand hygiene. Gloves should be used after proper hand hygiene has been done, and another hand hygiene routine must follow the removal of gloves from the hands.

Gowns and aprons

gowns and aprons are standard ppe used for protecting the skin and preventing clothing from getting soiled during procedures that are likely to cause splashing of blood and other body secretions. They must also be used when a contact-based infectious agent is suspected or has been diagnosed. Used gowns and aprons must be disposed of properly, and hand hygiene must be done after removal.

Masks

Masks and other eye protection equipment, such as goggles and face shields, are used as standard precautions during procedures that can result in splashes or sprays of blood and other body fluids. They are also used as a transmission-based precaution in situations where the patient is suspected to be infected with or has been diagnosed with an airborne or droplet-borne infectious agent.

Since simple masks are less expensive and often readily available, they are a standard precaution PPE that phlebotomist technicians can always incorporate for optimum protection and infection control. Other highly specialized surgical masks are strongly recommended as droplet-based transmission precautions. Masks are not recommended as efficient protective equipment for airborne transmission precaution. Instead, respirators should be used for optimum protection against airborne infections.

Eye Protection

Eye protection equipment such as goggles and face shields may be used as a standard precaution to protect the eyes from exposure to blood or other body fluids that may splash or spray during phlebotomy. They are also strongly recommended as a contact-based precautionary measure. They should be disposed of after each use, and hands should be thoroughly washed after they are disposed of.

Respirator

Respiratory protective equipment (RPE) is highly specialized PPE used as a precautionary measure against the inhalation of airborne infectious agents. RPE should only be used where adequate infection control cannot be achieved by any other means.

Respirators can be disposable or reusable. Disposable and single-use respirators are the most efficient for ensuring proper control of highly infectious airborne microorganisms.

Handling and Disposal of Sharp and Biohazardous Waste

Infection control measures are not complete without proper disposal of contaminated materials. These materials, when not properly disposed of, can pose a new risk of infection to anyone who may come in contact with them. Besides, many of the equipment used during phlebotomy, such as needles and lancets, are, on their own, dangerous, with the risk of punctures and cuts when not properly disposed of.

Biohazardous wastes include:

- Blood and blood products in any state, including fluids and materials that have been contaminated or saturated with blood.
- Pathological wastes, such as human anatomical parts in their containers.
- Cultures, stocks of infectious agents, and waste produced from biological
- Bedding/linens that have been saturated with blood and other bodily fluids.
- Vials and other containers used for storing blood, cultures, and other highly infectious solutions.
- Biotechnological and genetically altered product
- Used sharps.

Handling of Sharp Waste and Used PPE

Sharp waste, which includes needles, lancets, scalpels, and razors, is a potential hazard to healthcare workers, patients, and the general public. Not only can they cause punctures and injuries, but they can also transmit bloodborne diseases during such punctures.

Sharp waste should be disposed of immediately after use in designated sharp containers, also known as puncture-resistant containers. These containers must be clearly labeled to show their use, should be leak proof, and indeed puncture resistant.

Here are tips for managing and handling sharps up until they are ready to be finally disposed of, as recommended by the NCDC:

- Translucent puncture-proof containers should be used for the primary disposal of sharp waste. They should be available at easily accessible points in the healthcare environment.
- When using sharps, extreme care should be taken to avoid auto-inoculation.
- Needles should not be removed, bent, twisted, or manipulated in any form from syringes once they have been used. Used needles should, however, not be recapped before disposal.
- Used sharps should not be passed from one person to another. Each personnel should dispose of used sharps by themselves.
- It is important to know that needlestick injuries can also happen during disposal. It is, therefore, important for handling personnel to be experienced and remain mindful of all of their activities at all times.

Before final disposal, collected used needles can first be destroyed using a needle destroyer, disinfected, and be readied for final discarding by transferring them into a puncture-proof container. Disinfection can be done using 1% freshly prepared sodium hypochlorite solution (bleach).

Handling of Biohazardous Waste

Biohazardous wastes are materials contaminated with bodily fluids, such as blood, urine, feces, saliva, and mucus. These include all of the PPE used during phlebotomy, vials, and other equipment that are used for storing, transmitting and processing blood and other bodily fluids. When not properly disposed of, biohazardous waste poses a great risk of infection from microorganisms to healthcare workers, patients, non-healthcare workers working in healthcare environments, every other individual, animals, and even plants.

All materials contaminated with bodily fluids should be disposed of in biohazard bags or containers clearly labeled with a biohazard symbol. Bags must be leak proof and properly sealed before disposal.

Biohazardous wastes are dangerous sources of microorganism infection, whether or not they have been disinfected. Disinfecting or sterilizing some types of waste before disposal can be near impossible or uneconomical. It is, therefore, important they are handled and stored properly until they are completely disposed of.

When possible, however, waste bags should be autoclaved and treated to drastically reduce the risk of infections until they are finally disposed of.

Disposing of Sharp and Biohazardous Waste

It is important to carefully look into how biohazardous wastes and sharp wastes are finally disposed of once and for all. Certain disposal methods, such as burning, release harmful substances into the atmosphere that pose a further environmental threat.

It is therefore essential for healthcare facilities to have an efficient waste management section that factors in the proper disposal of high-risk waste and is in accordance with local and federal regulations for waste disposal.

At every point in the handling and disposal process, waste bins should be properly labeled using widely known words, letterings, and symbols to designate what each bin is for and what should go in which.

CHAPTER SUMMARY

- Infection control and safety are critical components of any medical procedure.

- Infection spreads through this definite chain:
  Agent ------------> Mode of transmission ------------> Susceptible host

- Agents are the microorganisms responsible for causing infections. They are classified as viruses, bacteria, fungi, and parasites.

- The portal of exit is the passageway through which an infectious agent leaves its reservoir or initial host.

- The mode of transmission is the specific way or medium that bears the infectious agent as it exits the reservoir. There are five important types of modes of transmission, which are: contact, airborne, droplet, common vehicle and vector-borne.

- The portal of entry offers an entry point for the infectious agent into the susceptible host.

- Infection control is essential at every point in the chain of infection to limit the risk of transmission of infectious agents from one individual to the other.

- Handwashing, medical asepsis, barrier protection, isolation, transmission-based precautions and use of PPE are standard precautions required of phlebotomy technicians.

- Sharp waste should be disposed of immediately after use in designated sharp containers, also known as puncture-resistant containers.

- Biohazardous wastes are materials contaminated with bodily fluids, such as blood, urine, feces, saliva, and mucus.

- All materials contaminated with bodily fluids should be disposed of in biohazard bags or containers clearly labeled with a biohazard symbol.

CHAPTER EIGHT: LEGAL CONSIDERATIONS

"It may seem a strange principle to enunciate as the very first requirement in a hospital that it should do the sick no harm."– Florence Nightingale

Legal considerations are needed in almost every sector, especially healthcare because healthcare places several people in vulnerable positions.

Fundamentally, healthcare places the patient in a vulnerable position to the actions or inactions of the healthcare personnel. However, caring for the sick also makes the healthcare personnel vulnerable to contracting several infectious diseases that can be hazardous to their health.

Therefore, the law must protect the patient receiving the care as well as the healthcare personnel delivering the care.

In taking samples, phlebotomists are exposed to infectious agents that can be easily transmitted through contact with blood and other specimens, needle prick injuries and patient contact.

To combat this, some special legislation has been made in the past.

1. NeedleStick Prevention Act: The Needlestick Safety and Prevention Act was passed by US Congress in 2001 as a revision to the then-existing Occupational Exposure to Bloodborne Pathogens standard. This revision resulted from the increased frequency of needlestick injuries to healthcare personnel in the United States. This update to OSHA's previous laws is reflected in 4 major areas:

Exposure Control Plan

The goal here is to limit or reduce the exposure of healthcare personnel to bloodborne pathogens. This is done by considering the innovations and technological advancements that can help reduce the exposure risk. This can be in the form of newly designed medical equipment that would reduce the use of needlesticks. It can also be in the form of using safer devices that are also effective in performing the functions. Such devices must be those that would not expose the patient or healthcare personnel to harm, would not go against medical principles, and would also reduce the likelihood of an exposure to a bloodborne pathogen through a contaminated sharp device.

Employee Input

Employers must obtain input from their employees that are in direct contact with patients and are at the highest risk of exposure. They should obtain input from them on safer medical devices and identify, evaluate and select effective engineering controls.

All employees included in this input should be across several sections of the hospital so that every section and situation of exposure that might be encountered in the workplace is well represented.

It is also expedient for all employers to document the way they obtained input from their employees, which can be by a list of employees and the method of input or other documents that might be used to show that responses were obtained from employees, e.g., minutes of meetings, surveys, etc.

Record Keeping

Employers are also required to keep an accurate record of employees who were exposed to blood or other infectious materials, as well as information on the device that was involved with the accident, the department where it happened, and a description of how the incident happened. In doing all this, the affected employee's information must be kept confidential.

Change of Definitions

Changes were made to some of the terms involving engineering controls:

- 'Engineering controls' was made more specific and allowed to include all the control measures that can either reduce or isolate any hazard in the workplace (e.g., sharp disposal box or self-sheathing needles). It was also extended to mean needleless systems and other sharps injury protections and specified that these must be used where necessary.
- 'Sharps with engineered sharp injury protections' is a new term that was added, and it refers to all non-needle sharps or needle devices that contain safety features that are built-in or fitted. Examples include shielded or retracting catheters, needles that retract inside a syringe after use, etc.
- 'Needleless systems' was also introduced as a new term. It refers to devices that could be an alternative to using needles on various procedures to reduce the risk of injury from contaminated sharps. Some of these examples include IV medication systems that utilize non-needle connections or jet injection systems that deliver fluids and medications under the skin.

2. The Health Insurance Portability and Accountability Act (HIPAA) places demands on physicians to ensure the protection of electronically stored protected health information (PHI) of patients, by using all possible safeguards. These safeguards include administrative, technical and physical methods to ensure that the confidentiality, and integrity of PHI is maintained.

- Administrative safeguards deal with the policies and administrative actions that regulate the entire process of obtaining and storing PHI, from the development to implementation stages. All of these must be done to ensure that PHI is confidential. It includes training, procedures, and policies to determine who has access or not.

- Physical safeguards are concerned with both physical and electronic structures. PHI and computers storing PHI, must be kept from unauthorized access using barriers like security systems, passwords, codes that are only available to authorized personnel.
- Technical safeguards are concerned with the technical aspects of the program and how it runs that ensure that PHI is truly secure and confidential.

3. Patient's Bill of Rights lists the rights and responsibilities of a patient that are consistent with law. Some are listed below. A patient has the right to:

- Receive treatment without any form of discrimination.

- Receive emergency treatment if needed.

- Complete information on the diagnosis and the treatment of the condition.

- Review their own medical records without charge.

- Accept or refuse treatment.

Other legal considerations include:

- Informed consent refers to the consent a patient gives for performing a procedure with a full understanding of its benefits, risks, alternatives and expected results. A phlebotomist must always ensure that a patient gives informed consent before performing any procedure.
- Patient confidentiality is extremely important in the management of patient information and is well addressed by the HIPAA. Patient confidentiality must be strictly maintained throughout the care of the patient. Information should only be disclosed on a need-to-know basis; that is, people who would not need the information for the direct or indirect care of the patient do not need to know about the condition of the patient.

- Negligence refers to the failure of a person who is supposed to give a specific level of care to a patient, resulting in harm or loss to the patient. It is the failure to perform the level of care that anyone with the level of training and in the same circumstances would give. It has four elements which are Duty (Duty of care), Derelict (means a breach of the duty of care), Direct cause (An injury or legally recognized assault that results from a breach of duty of care), and Damage (which refers to the wrongful action that must have resulted in the injury or harm)

- Tort refers to the inappropriate or wrong action that a person performs, which causes injury to another person. In the clinic, these can be battery, invasion of privacy, defamation of character through written(libel) or slander (spoken form)

- Good Samaritan Law is a law that protects healthcare personnel, allowing them to render any healthcare service within the scope of their training in an accident or sudden injury without the fear of being charged for negligence.

CHAPTER SUMMARY

- Legal considerations are needed in almost every sector, especially healthcare, because healthcare places several people in vulnerable positions.

- Some special legislation has been made in the past.
  - NeedleStick Prevention Act: The Needlestick Safety and Prevention Act was passed by US Congress in 2001 as a result of the increased frequency of needlestick injuries to healthcare personnel in the United States.
  - The Health Insurance Portability and accountability Act (HIPAA): The HIPAA places demands on physicians to ensure the protection of electronically stored protected health information (PHI) of patients, by using all possible safeguards.
  - Patient's Bill of Rights: The Patient Bill of Right lists the rights and responsibilities of a patient that are consistent with law.

- Others include:

  - Informed consent: Refers to the consent a patient gives for performing a procedure with a full understanding of its benefits, risks, alternatives and expected results.

- o Patient confidentiality: Information should only be disclosed on a need-to-know basis, that is, people who would not need the information for the direct or indirect care of the patient do not need to know about the condition of the patient.
- o Negligence: Refers to the failure of a person who is supposed to give a specific level of care to a patient, resulting in harm or loss to the patient.
- o Tort: Refers to the inappropriate or wrong action that a person performs, which causes injury to another person.
- o Good Samaritan Law: This law protects healthcare personnel, allowing them to render any healthcare service within the scope of their training in an accident or sudden injury without the fear of being charged for negligence.

QUESTIONS

1. Which is the most preferred vein for venipuncture?

A. Median Cubital Vein

B. Cephalic Vein

C. Basilic Vein

D. Great Saphenous Vein

2. Why should tortuous veins be avoided in a venipuncture?

A. Cordlike nature

B. Prone to infection

C. Seen in diabetics

D. Lymphedema

3. A 55-year-old man is directed to you for a venipuncture by the doctor. He is a known diabetic with very difficult veins. Which of the following areas do you want to avoid at all costs?

A. Arm

B. Forearm

C. Foot

D. None of the above.

4. Which is not a chamber in the heart?

A. Left Auricle

B. Left Atrium

C. Right Ventricle

D. Tricuspid sinus

5. What type of blood flows through the pulmonary artery?

A. Oxygenated blood

B. Deoxygenated blood

C. All of the above

D. None of the above

6. Which of the following statements is false?

A. The systemic circulation receives blood from the pulmonary circulation

B. The systemic circulation takes oxygenated blood from the left ventricle to the aorta

C. The pulmonary vein takes blood away from the heart

D. The pulmonary vein takes blood to the heart

7. One of the following is not part of the 3 layers of the heart

A. Endocardium

B. Mesocardium

C. Myocardium

D. Epicardium

8. What three branches are formed at the aortic arch?

A. Brachiocephalic trunk, right common carotid artery, right subclavian artery

B. Visceral and parietal arterial branches

C. Inferior and superior mesenteric arteries, renal arteries, iliac arteries

D. Brachiocephalic trunk, left common carotid artery, left subclavian artery

9. Superficial veins of the lower limb include the following except

A. Great saphenous vein

B. Small saphenous vein

C. Popliteal vein

D. None of the above

10. What do both arteries and veins have in common?

A. Valves

B. Use muscle compressions to push blood

C. Both have walls

D. Both are easily distensible

11. What are the components of blood?

A. Formed elements and white blood cells

B. Formed elements and water

C. Plasma and formed elements

D. All of the above

12. What is the shape of erythrocytes?

A. Cuboid

B. Circular

C. Ellipsoid

D. Formless

13. Which is the most common type of leukocyte?

A. Neutrophils

B. Monocytes

C. Lymphocytes

D. Macrophages

14. Which of the following is the first responder when there is an infection?

A. Monocytes

B. Lymphocytes

C. Basophils

D. Neutrophils

15. Which type of white blood cell has a bilobed nucleus and is implicated in allergies?

A. Basophils

B. Eosinophils

C. Monocytes

D. Neutrophils

16. The largest type of white blood cells are

A. Eosinophils

B. Basophils

C. Monocytes

D. Lymphocytes

17. A patient developed an allergy after a medication was given for the first time, with an accompanying skin reaction. Which of the following is most likely implicated?

A. Basophil

B. Eosinophil

C. Neutrophil

D Lymphocyte

18. Thrombocytes have a life span of

A. 120 days

B. 9 - 12 days

C. 2 weeks

D. 2 months

19. Which of the following is not a characteristic of platelets?

A. Adhesion

B. Aggregation

C. Coarseness

D. Agglutination

20. Thrombocytes are formed in the

A. Liver

B. Plasma

C. Bone marrow

D. Thymus

Patient preparation

21. Which of the following does not need to be filled in a requisition form?

A. Patient Name

B. Patient's relative's name

C. Requesting physician

D. DOB of patient

22. You want to take a CBC sample from a patient who is comatose. What do you do to ensure proper identification?

A. Check the requisition order and label the sample with the same name.

B. Check the bracelet and ask the caregiver/relative for the full name to confirm.

C. Ask the patient to spell their full name.

D. All of the above

23. A 65 year old woman had a right mastectomy a year ago. Where would you take her samples from?

A. Right leg

B. Right forearm

C. Left forearm

D. Left leg

24. What is the most important factor to consider in taking a sample to test for cortisol levels?

A. Fasting

B. Time of the day

C. Urgency

D. Age of the patient

25. Which of the following factors would affect the venipuncture site in a patient who has had a previous mastectomy?

A. Fasting

B. Fistulas

C. Timing

D. Edema

26. A 55-year-old man presented to the clinic and collapsed on the floor while he was being attended to. Samples need to be taken for tests. What type of consent would be used here?

A. Informed consent

B. Express consent

C. Implied consent

D. None

27. Why do phlebotomists avoid arteriovenous fistulas?

A. Prone to bleeding

B. Prone to infection

C. Aesthetically unpleasing

D. All of the above

28. Which of the following actions is not part of patient preparation?

A. Asking about fasting state

B. Asking about latex allergy

C. Confirming the test for taking the blood sample

D. Writing patient's names on sample tubes before sample collection

29. What antiseptic would you use to clean the selected phlebotomy site for a lipid panel?

A. Povidone-iodine

B. 20% isopropyl alcohol

C. 70% isopropyl alcohol

D. Clean water

30. Which equipment is useful in taking samples from very tiny veins?

A. Tourniquet

B. Gloves

C. Vacutainer bottle

D. Butterfly

31. Which of the following is not part of the process of drawing blood?

A. Greeting the patient

B. Explaining the procedure to the patient

C. Recapping the needle before disposal

D. Palpating the vein

32. At what angle should the bevel be inserted into the vein?

A. 20 - 40 degrees

B. 60 degrees

C. 15 - 30 degrees

D. 90 degrees

33. How long should the tourniquet be in place?

A. 5 minutes

B. 1 minute

C. 3 minutes

D. None of the above

34. What cover should come before the red in the order of draw?

A. Blue

B. Green

C. Lavender

D. Gray

35. Which of the following bottles should be filled last?

A. Blood culture

B. Plain bottle

C. Oxalate/Fluoride bottles

D. EDTA bottles.

36. In which order should the following samples be taken: CBC, coagulation studies, fasting blood glucose fluoride, blood culture

A. Blood culture, coagulation studies, CBC, fasting blood glucose.

B. Blood culture, CBC, coagulation studies, fasting blood glucose

C. Fasting blood glucose, CBC, coagulation studies, blood culture

D. CBC, fasting blood glucose, coagulation studies, blood culture

37. How would you prevent a hematoma from forming after taking a sample?

A. Release the tourniquet earlier

B. Tell the patient to bend the arm

C. Apply pressure with the tip of your thumb

D. None of the above

38. When should you call for help if bleeding does not subside?

A. After 2 mins

B. After 5 minutes

C. After 8 minutes

D. After an hour

39. Which of the following is not correct in performing a venipuncture?

A. patient should make a fist

B. Allow the alcohol on the venipuncture site to dry before inserting the needle

C. Gathering all your equipment after cleaning the site

D. Samples should be taken in order of flow

40. What is the length of the vacutainer needle commonly needed for venipuncture?

A. 1.0, 1.5 inches

B. 2.0, 3.0 inches

C. 2.0, 2.5 inches

D. All of the above

41. What is the diameter of the needle that is commonly used in venipuncture?

A. 10 - 15 gauge

B. 16 - 23 gauge

C. > 23 gauge

D. < 6 gauge

42. When a vein collapses, what is the best solution?

A. Reinsert the needle into the vein

B. Adjust the angle of the needle

C. Tighten the tourniquet

D. Look for another vein to get the sample

43. What should you do when you completely miss the vein during a venipuncture?

A. Remove the needle completely and look for another vein

B. Redirect the needle with a gloved hand

C. Slowly elevate the angle of the needle

D. All of the above

44. What is the solution for a patient who has had venipuncture done so many times, they are now uncooperative?

A. Explaining patiently and reassuring the patient

B. Forcefully take the sample

C. Leave the patient alone

D. Avoid such patients

45. A 60 year old woman had two mastectomies done on the right and the left. The last one was done a year ago on the left side. Where would you draw her samples from?

A. Her right forearm

B. Her left forearm

C. Her foot as a last resort

D. None of the above

46. What method is usually used to take a sample from a pediatric patient?

A. Forcefully

B. Distracting them with a role play

C. Putting them to sleep

D. None of the above

47. When is the butterfly infusion set useful?

A. Really small veins

B. Pediatric patients

C. Elderly patients

D All of the above

48. Which of the following is most suitable for taking samples from infants when just a little blood sample is required?

A. Venipuncture

B. Dermal puncture

C. Butterfly infusion set

D. All of the above

49. What is the maximum recommended depth for heel puncture in infants?

A. 1.0mm

B. 2.0mm

C. 3.0mm

D. 4.0mm

50. Which finger is used for dermal puncture in adults?

A. Any finger can be used

B. 2nd finger

C. 3rd finger

D. B and C

51. One major difference between dermal puncture and venipuncture is

A. Sites used

B. Prewarming

C. Technique

D. All of the above

52. Order of draw for puncture specimen?

A. Lavender, tube without additives, tube with additives

B. Lavender, tube with additives, tube without additives

C. Tube with additives, tube without additives, lavender

D. None of the above

53. Which of the following is not used in dermal puncture?

A. 70% isopropyl alcohol

B. Povidone-iodine

C. Gloves

D. Towel

54. Dermal puncture is not suitable for one of the following

A. ESR

B. Blood glucose

C. CBC

D. Neonatal bilirubin

55. Which complication results from capillary rupture from prolonged tourniquet use?

A. Phlebitis

B. Thrombophlebitis

C. Petechiae

D. Wounds

56. One way to avoid a needle prick injury is to:

A. Recap used needles with great caution

B. Avoid needles as much as possible

C. Never recap used needles

D. All of the above

57. Inflammation of the vein and clot formation is known as

A. Phlebitis

B. Petechiae

C. Thrombophlebitis

D. Septicemia

58. What are the sites for dermal punctures in infants?

A. Medial and lateral regions

B. Medial and lateral regions of the plantar surface of the foot

C. Medial and lateral regions of the dorsum

D. All of the above.

59. What is quality assurance?

A. Protocols put in place to ensure a process goes smoothly

B. Established systems to ensure a service meets the specified requirement

C. Patient preparation

D. Patient reassurance

60. Which of the following errors happens after sample collection?

A. Incorrect patient positioning

B. Interference of medication

C. No fast for samples require fasting

D. Failure of serum-cell preparation

61. Hemolysis is an error that occurs

A. Before sample collection

B. During sample collection

C. After sample collection

D. All of the above.

62. How to protect light-sensitive samples?

A. Use dark sample bottles in the collection

B. Wrap with gauze

C. Wrap in aluminum foil

D. None of the above

63. Which of the following should be stored with ice packs immediately after storage?

A. Bilirubin test

B. Porphyrin

C. Arterial blood gasses

D. Samples for direct Coombs test

64. Which samples should be stored at higher temperatures?

A. Beta-carotene

B. Lactic acid

C. Ammonia

D. Samples for direct Coombs test

65. What is tested in a 2 hrs postprandial test?

A. Fasting glucose is compared to glucose 2hrs after a meal

B. Random blood glucose is compared with 2hrs after a meal

C. Fasting blood glucose is compared at 2hrs interval

D. All of the above

66. An example of a substance that requires a timed specimen due to diurnal variation is

A. Water

B. Cortisol

C. Hemoglobin

D. Digoxin

67. What specimen is taken to identify the presence of microorganisms in the blood?

A. PKU

B. Electrolytes

C. Blood cultures

D. Electrolytes

68. When are trough-level samples taken in drug monitoring?

A. An hour after the first dose

B. 30 mins before the first dose

C. Two hours after drug administration before the peak

D. 30 mins after the first dose

69. One precaution for blood culture samples is to

A. Transport them to the lab immediately, as they are affected by cold

B. Transport them to the lab the following day

C. Transport them to the lab immediately, as samples are affected by temperature and passage of time

D. All of the above

70. Samples for PKU are taken from where in the newborn?

A. 3rd or 4th finger

B. 2nd or 3rd finger

C. Heel

D. All of the above.

71. Which of the following tests are not analyzed in the hematology section of a clinical laboratory?

A. CBC

B. Toxicology

C. ESR

D. Peripheral blood film

72. What test is used to evaluate the potency of the intrinsic pathway?

A. APTT

B. PT

C. TT

D. Reticulocyte count

73. What test is used to evaluate the potency of the extrinsic pathway?

A. APTT

B. PT

C. TT

D. Peripheral blood film

74. What is or are identified and quantified in the chemical section of the lab?

A. Chemical reactions

B. Decaying time

C. Half-life

D. Speed

75. Tests that are carried out in the chemistry section include

A. Electrophoresis

B. Immunochemistry

C. None of the above

D. All of the above

76. The liver profile test comprises the following except

A. ALP

B. ALT

C. ADT

D. GGT

77. Which of the following is not a common sample used to detect classes of drugs or poisons in a person's body?

A. Sweat

B. Blood

C. Urine

D. Earlobe

78. Commonly transmitted viruses through needlestick injuries are

A. HIV, HEP A

B. HIV, HEP B

C. HEP A, HEP B, HIV

D. HEP C, HEP A

79. Which section checks for chances of acceptance or rejection of body tissue in organ transplants?

A. Hematology

B. Chemistry

C. Blood bank

D. Serology/immunology

80. Which section is involved in identifying parasites in the body?

A. Microbiology

B. Hematology

C. Chemistry

D. Serology/immunology

81. What are autoimmune disorders?

A. The body produces antibodies against foreign bodies

B. The body produces antibodies against transplanted organs

C. The body produces antibodies against its own organs

D. Disorders characterized by hypopigmentation

82. What are immunodeficiency disorders?

A. Disorders that excessively strengthen the deficient areas of the immune system

B. Disorders that weaken the immune system

C. Opportunistic infections

D. B and C

83. What section of the laboratory is heavily involved in infection control?

A. Hematology

B. Serology/Immunology

C. Microbiology

D. Chemistry

84. What test is important when a patient is experiencing a fever of unknown origin?

A. CBC

B. Electrolyte

C. Culture and sensitivity

D. ESR

85. Which specimen is not routinely used in microbiology?

A. Urine

B. Sputum

C. Blood

D. Hair

86. One drawback of some cultures is

A. Not specific enough

B. Not useful

C. Results can take a longer time

D. None of the above

87. Macroscopic properties of urine that are examined include:

A. Casts

B. Glucose

C. Color

D. Microorganisms

88. What is the danger of leaving the tourniquet on for more than two minutes?

A. Hemolysis

B. Hemoconcentration

C. Hemostasis

D. Homeostasis

89. Tests that can be performed on urine include the following except

A. Microscopy

B. Culture and sensitivity

C. Chemical examinations

D. None of the above

90. An example of diseases that can be diagnosed from the urine include

A. Diabetes insipidus

B. Pulmonary TB

C. HIV

D. All of the above

91. The NeedleStick Prevention Act was passed by Congress in

A. 1999

B. 2000

C. 2001

D. 2010

92. Which of the following is an area of the NeedleStick Prevention Act

A. Record keeping

B. Change of definitions

C. Employee Input

D. All of the above

93. A nurse is telling a cleaner in the health facility from another ward about the patient status of a patient in her ward. What right of the patient is being breached?

A. Informed consent

B. Implied consent

C. Patient confidentiality

D. Negligence

94. A woman who is too weak to speak needs a sample to be taken for CBC. After explaining to her, she does not say anything but stretches her arm to you. What kind of consent is this?

A. Implied consent

B. Expressed consent

C. No consent

D. Negligence

95. What is tort?

A. Going ahead to perform a procedure without asepsis and causing infection to the patient

B. Failure to take a sample when a patient is ready

C. Inability to obtain blood from a vein while taking a sample

D. All of the above

96. What law allows healthcare personnel to render healthcare service within the scope of their training at an accident site without fear of being charged with negligence?

A. HIPAA

B. Good Samaritan law

C. Bill of rights

D. Advance directive

97. A nurse is being charged with negligence against one of her patients. What does this mean?

A. She did not give the expected level of care

B. Patient suffered harm or injury because she did not give the expected level of care

C. She committed a wrong act

D. All of the above

98. What are the elements of negligence

A. Duty, derelict, direct cause, damage

B. Damage control, duty, direct, derelict

C. Duty, direct cause, damage control loss

D. Damage control, duty care, derelict, direct cause.

99. What is the breach of duty of care?

A. Duty

B. Damage

C. Damage control

D. Derelict

100. How much information does a phlebotomist need about the patient's status?

A. Every important detail of the patient

B. Everything the doctor knows

C. As much as is important to perform their role as a phlebotomist

D. None of the above

101. Immunity can be classified into:

A. Acquired and Innate

B. Acquired and T-cell

C. T-cell and B-cell

D. All of the above

102. Two classifications of immunity include:

A. T and B-cell mediated

B. Cell-mediated and T-cell mediated

C. Humoral and B-cell mediated

D. A-cell and B-cell mediated.

103. What is the first line of defense of the body against invading pathogens?

A. Acquired

B. B-cell

C. T-cell

D. Innate

104. Phagocytosis exhibited by neutrophils and macrophages is an example of

A. Acquired immunity

B. B-cell mediated immunity

C. Innate immunity

D. None of the above

105. Which WBC mediates acquired immunity?

A. Neutrophil

B. Macrophage

C. Lymphocyte

D. Eosinophils

106. Which of the following is true about cellular immunity?

A. Mediated by B-cells

B. Mediated by T-cells

C. No antibody production

D. B and C

107. Which of the following is true about humoral immunity?

A. Mediated by B-cells

B. Involves antigen detection

C. There is antibody production

D. All of the above

108. What is opsonization?

A. Optimization of blood cells for transfusion

B. Process of antibodies marking pathogenic cells

C. Destruction of pathogenic cells

D. All of the above

109. Which of the following are the stages involved in hemostasis?

A. Vasoconstriction, platelet plug formation, blood coagulation

B. Vasoconstriction, homeostasis, serum coagulation, plug sealing

C. Vasodilatation, platelet aggregation, plug sealing, wound closure

D. None of the above

110. What is secreted by the platelets after adherence?

A. ADP

B. ATP

C. ALP

D. GGT

111. What are the stages of the coagulation cascade?

A. Formation of prothrombin factor activator

B. Conversion of prothrombin to thrombin

C. Conversion of fibrinogen to fibrin

D. All of the above

112. What is the process of removing the clot from inside the blood vessel called?

A. Fibrinogenolysis

B. Fibrinization

C. Clot breakdown

D. Fibrinolysis

113. Which of the following statements is incorrect?

A. Vasoconstriction in hemostasis is systemic

B. Platelets exhibit adherence and aggregation

C. Serotonin is also secreted by platelets

D. Fibrinolysis occurs after clot formation

114. What is the function of the Von Willebrand Factor?

A. Facilitates aggregation

B. Facilitates adherence

C. Facilitates serotonin secretion

D. All of the above

115. Is phlebotomy the same as venipuncture?

A. No, phlebotomy is a field and a discipline, venipuncture is a procedure.

B. Yes, they are the same

C. Venipuncture is a field, phlebotomy is a procedure

D. None of the above

116. What type of vein would you most likely see in a patient taking chemotherapy?

A. Collapsed veins

B. AV fistula

C. Sclerosed veins

D. Difficult veins

117. Which of the following should be avoided when taking blood samples?

A. Pediatric patients

B. Elderly patients

C. Patients that have diabetes mellitus

D. Arm with IV fluid running

118. What bottle is suitable for glucose tolerance test samples?

A. Gray top

B. Light blue top

C. Green top

D. Red top

119. Which sample bottle contains heparin?

A. Red top

B. Blue top

C. Green top

D. Gray top

120. What is contained in the yellow top bottle?

A. SPS

B. EDTA

C. Fluoride oxalate

D. No additive

121. One of the following is not a reason why it is essential to follow proper infection control and safety procedures during phlebotomy:

A. To minimize the risk of infection transmission

B. For ensuring the safety of patients and healthcare workers

C. To ensure the patient gets well soon

D. None of the above

122. Which of these rightly describes what an agent is?

A. An individual who carries infectious microorganisms and is responsible for transmitting these microorganisms to others

B. The medium that transmits microorganisms from one point to the other

C. Contaminated equipment that serves as a potential source of infection

D. Disease-causing microorganisms

123. Which of these is the phlebotomist technician responsible for?

A. Treating infection in patients after they have been diagnosed

B. Diagnosing the patient for likely infections before phlebotomy

C. Ensuring the patient wears the right personal protective equipment before phlebotomy

D. None of the above

124. If a patient on whom phlebotomy is to be carried out, is diagnosed with a highly infectious airborne microorganism, which one of the following should be done?

A. Utilize transmission-based precautions with standard precautions

B. Utilize standard precautions alone

C. Utilize transmission-based precautions alone

D. Ensure the patient is first of all treated and then utilize standard precautions.

125. Which of the following is not true about standard precautions?

A. They are cheaper alternatives to transmission-based precautions

B. They cannot be used alongside transmission-based precautions

C. They should not be used when a patient is suspected to be infected, but has not yet been diagnosed

D. None of the above

126. Infection to the phlebotomist technician can be prevented by:

A. Asking the patient to wash their hands before phlebotomy is done

B. The phlebotomist technician putting on personal protective equipment

C. Treating the patient for infection before phlebotomy

D. All of the above

127. Which of these rightly describes what a droplet is?

A. Agent

B. Mode of transmission

C. Medium

D. Portal of exit

128. Portal of exit is to reservoir, while portal of entry is to:

A. Microorganism

B. Medium

C. Susceptible host

D. Agent

129. Which of the following statements is true?

A. A host is a potential reservoir

B. The host transmits infection to the reservoir

C. The reservoir is a potential host

D. None of the above

130. Which of the following represents the correct order of the chain of infection?

A. Agent ---> Portal of transmission ---> Susceptible host

B. Agent ---> Portal of Exit ---> Portal of Entry ---> Reservoir

C. Agent ---> Mode of transmission ---> Susceptible host

D. Agent ---> Reservoir ---> Portal of Entry ---> Susceptible host

131. There are _____ modes of transmission

A. 5

B. 6

C. 3

D. 4

132. The alimentary canal is to _____ as broken skin is to _____

A. Susceptible host, reservoir

B. Mode of transmission, medium

C. Portal of entry, portal of exit

D. Portal of exit, portal of entry

133. _____ are the routine activities that must be carried out to achieve a basic level of infection prevention and control

A. Minimum precautions

B. Standard precautions

C. Infection control

D. Transmission-based precautions

134. Standard precautions are recommended because

A. They are affordable

B. All humans potentially harbor infectious agents

C. They are quick and easy to implement

D. All of the above

135. Which of the following is not considered a standard precaution?

A. Use of gloves

B. Hand washing

C. Use of respirators

D. Disinfection of used equipment

136. _____ is the act of destroying microorganisms and infectious agents after they've let the body.

A. Disinfection

B. Waste disposal

C. Biohazardous waste

D. Medical asepsis

137. Household bleach in water solution for disinfection should be mixed in what ratio?

A.1:10

B. 2:5

C. 3:10

D. 1:5

138. Disinfectants can be used for washing hands as well as for disinfecting equipment

A. True

B. False

C. Maybe

D. I don't know

139. Gloves, masks, face shields, and goggles are all examples of what?

A. PPE

B. Barrier protection

C. All of the above

D. None of the above

140. How should a used needle be disposed of?

A. Removed from the syringe and placed in a puncture-proof container

B. Recapped after used and placed in a puncture-proof container

C. Disposed into the nearest wastepaper basket

D. Left uncapped after use and placed in a puncture-proof container

141. Transmission-based precautions are used when?

A. The patient can afford to pay for them

B. Standard precautions alone will not suffice

C. There is no standard precaution PPE available

D. As a replacement for standard precautions

142. There are _____ distinct categories of transmission-based precautions.

A. 2

B. 3

C. 4

D. 5

143. Which of the following is not true of gloves?

A. They can be reused

B. There is no need to wash hands after using gloves

C. They are an example of transmission-based precautions

D. None of the above

144. Biohazardous wastes include all the following except:

A. Used sharps

B. Puncture-proof containers

C. Bodily fluids

D. Beddings/linens that have been contaminated with blood

145. Which of the following is a proper practice for disposing of biohazardous waste?

A. Properly labeling waste containers

B. Using a wastepaper bin for disposing of used needles

C. Recapping used needles before they are disposed of

D. Options A and C

146. Autoclaving is the process of

A. sealing biohazardous waste in sterile bags

B. sterilizing used equipment using bleach

C. sterilizing used equipment using steam

D. destroying needles and syringes before they are disposed of

147. Biohazardous wastes are essentially:

A. Wastes that are potentially contaminated with infectious agents

B. Wastes that contain harmful chemicals

C. Non-degradable waste

D. All of the above

148. Which of the following is not classified as biohazardous waste?

A. Human anatomical parts

B. Vials that have been used for storing body fluids

C. Chemicals

D. Genetically altered products

149. Eye protection PPE includes all of the following except:

A. Face shields

B. Respirators

C. Goggles

D. None of the above

150. One of the following is not true of barrier protection PPE.

A. They are strictly transmission-based precautions

B. They protect from splashes and sprays

C. Some of them are reusable

D. Face shields and gloves are examples of barrier protectors

ANSWERS

1. A. Median cubital vein.

The median cubital vein is the most preferred venipuncture vein because it is easily accessible, usually straight and superficially placed in the forearm. It is also usually wide enough to accommodate the needle and not so close to other delicate structures like nerves or arteries, which are usually deep.

2. B. Prone to infection.

Tortuous veins are not straight and can make the process of obtaining the sample difficult. They are also very prone to infection and can produce altered or incorrect results.

3. C. Foot.

Veins in the lower limb are used only as a last resort because of their increased vulnerability to clot formation. Furthermore, this patient is a known diabetic, and injuries to the foot can result in diabetic foot disease. Therefore, the forearm is the most preferred area for venipuncture.

4. D. Tricuspid sinus.

The four chambers in the heart are the left auricle/atrium, the left ventricle, the right auricle/atrium, and the right ventricle. The tricuspid valve is the valve between the right auricle/atrium and the right ventricle. It ensures unidirectional blood flow by preventing regurgitation from the right ventricle into the right auricle.

5. B. Deoxygenated blood.

Deoxygenated blood flows from the right ventricle to the lungs for oxygenation through the pulmonary artery. This artery is the only artery in the body that carries deoxygenated blood.

6. C. The pulmonary vein takes blood away from the heart.

All veins take blood to the heart, including the pulmonary vein.

7. B. Mesocardium.

The 3 layers of the heart are the endocardium, the myocardium and the epicardium.

8. D. Brachiocephalic trunk, left common carotid artery, left subclavian artery.

From the heart, blood flows into the aorta, which then forms the aortic arch, which gives off 3 branches that supply the head and part of the upper limbs. They are the brachiocephalic trunk (largest), left common carotid artery and the left subclavian artery.

9. C. Popliteal vein.

Examples of superficial veins in the lower limb include the great and small saphenous veins, which both arise from the dorsal venous arch of the foot. The popliteal vein is a deep vein.

10. C. Both have walls.

Veins can be easily compressed because they have thinner walls and larger lumina than arteries. Since they are easily distensible, they allow the use of muscle compressions to push blood forward.

11. C. Plasma and formed elements.

12. C. Ellipsoid.

RBCs are ellipsoid in shape.

13. A. Neutrophils.

Neutrophils are the most prevalent type of leucocyte, forming between 40 and 70% of the total leucocyte population.

14. D. Neutrophils.

Neutrophils are usually the first responders when there is an infection.

15. A. Basophils.

Basophils are white blood cells with a bilobed nucleus. They are involved in allergic reactions in which they release histamine.

16. C. Monocytes.

Monocytes are the largest type of white blood cells. They also lack granules in their cytoplasm and have a nucleus that is either central or pushed to one corner of the cell. Once they get into tissues, they become macrophages which are involved in phagocytosis. They represent about 3 - 8% of the total white blood cells count in the body.

17. B. Eosinophil.

Eosinophils: These are involved in attacking foreign bodies that have been labeled by antibody molecules. They are also implicated in allergies and skin reactions. They form about 1 - 3% of the body's total white blood cells count.

18. B. 9 - 12 days.

Platelets are also known as thrombocytes. They are minute, anucleated bodies that are formed in the bone marrow. They are usually between 140000 - 400000 per microliter of blood and typically live for about 9 - 12 days.

19. C. Coarseness.

Platelets have the following properties: adhesion, aggregations, and agglutination, but not coarseness.

20. C. Bone marrow.

Thrombocytes (platelets) are minute, anucleated bodies that are formed in the bone marrow. They are adhesive, aggregate easily and agglutinate. These features are very important to the functions that they perform.

21. B. Patient relative name.

A requisition form should contain: Patient's name in full, patient's hospital ID number, government issued ID card, date of birth and sex of the patient, the full name of the requesting physician, the sample to be collected, that is blood, the test for which the sample is meant for. A patient's relative's name is not needed in a requisition form.

22. B. Check the bracelet and ask the caregiver/relative for the full name to confirm.

Since the patient is unconscious, you cannot get a response from the patient. Therefore, check the patient's bracelet, and then ask the relative/caregiver/nurse for the name and ensure they match with what is on the requisition form.

23. C. Left forearm.

The contralateral limb should be used in patients who have done a mastectomy on one side. If a patient has had more than one mastectomy, the limb contralateral to the last site should be used.

24. B. Time of the day.

Some tests are better done in the morning, when their levels in the blood are optimal, so that an accurate result can be obtained of the function of the substance. A good example of this is cortisol, which exhibits diurnal variation and is at peak levels are attained early in the morning, with a steady decline throughout the day.

25. D. Edema.

When there is edema in the upper limb especially, there is a high possibility of incorrect results. Patients who have had a mastectomy on one side usually have edema on the affected side.

26. C. Implied consent.

Implied consent is given by an action. Since the patient is not able to speak for himself and there is no relative or caregiver around or any advance directive given, then the patient can be treated on implied consent, that being in the hospital at that moment for treatment implies that the patient has agreed to whatever needs to be done to treat them according to standard healthcare practices.

27. B. Prone to infection.

Fistulas are arteriovenous connections and should be avoided in venipuncture as they can lead to infection.

28. D. Writing patient's names on sample tubes before sample collection.

Patient names should be written on sample bottles after collection, not before collection.

29. C. 70% isopropyl alcohol.

The most common antiseptic that is used is 70% isopropyl alcohol. Povidone iodine is used for swabs if the sample to be taken is for blood culture.

30. D. Butterfly.

Butterfly/winged infusion sets are useful in pediatric or elderly patients or generally small veins.

31. C. Recapping the needle before disposal.

Needles should not be recapped after use. Discard the used needle and syringes into the biohazard sharps container.

32. C. 15 - 30 degrees.

Insert the needle with the bevel turned upwards at an angle of 15 to 30 degrees to the surface of the arm.

33. B. 1 minute.

Once blood flow has been established, the tourniquet should not be kept in place for more than two minutes. This is to prevent hemoconcentration of the samples collected.

34. A. Blue.

The correct order of draw, as stated by the National Healthcareer Association, includes:

1. Blood culture bottles or vials
2. Sodium citrate bottles (blue cover)
3. Serum tubes or plain bottles (without clot activator) (red covers)
4. Heparin bottles (green cover)
5. EDTA bottles (lavender cover)
6. Oxalate/Fluoride bottles (gray cover).

35. C. Oxalate/fluoride bottles.

The correct order of draw, as stated by the National Healthcareer Association, includes:

1. Blood culture bottles or vials
2. Sodium citrate bottles (blue cover)
3. Serum tubes or plain bottles (without clot activator) (red covers)
4. Heparin bottles (green cover)

5. EDTA bottles (lavender cover)

6. Oxalate/Fluoride bottles (gray cover).

36. A. Blood culture, coagulation studies, CBC, fasting blood glucose.

Blood culture - Blood culture bottles or vials

Coagulation studies - blue top

CBC - EDTA (lavender)

Fasting blood glucose - Oxalate/fluoride bottles (gray cover)

According to the order of draw, that is the correct order.

37. D. None of the above.

To prevent hematoma, pressure should be applied with a sterile gauze over the venipuncture site, not just with the tip of a thumb.

38. C. After 8 minutes.

Excessive bleeding: Certain patients might have disease conditions or be on medications that do not allow bleeding to stop in time. Bleeding can also result if the needle is pushed into an artery. The phlebotomist should call for help if blood flow does not stop after a total of 8 minutes.

39. C. Gathering all your equipment after cleaning the site.

All equipment should have been gathered before cleaning the site. Assembly of needed materials should be one of the first steps to performing the procedure.

40. A. 1.0, 1.5 inches.

Vacutainer needles come in different sizes and lengths, but the 1.0-inch and 1.5-inch-length needles are commonly used. They are single use.

41. B. 16 - 23 gauge.

Needle diameters are arranged in such a way that the higher the number, the narrower the gauges. So, a 23-gauge is narrower than a 20-gauge needle.

42. D. Look for another vein to get the sample.

A collapsed vein is very difficult to access blood from. Hence just find another vein.

43. B. Redirect the needle with a gloved hand.

The vein might be completely missed upon introducing the needle. To fix this, examine the position of the vein and the needle with a gloved finger and slowly redirect it.

44. A. Explainingpatiently and reassuring the patient.

45. A. Her right forearm.

The contralateral limb should be used in patients who have done a mastectomy on one side. If a patient has had more than one mastectomy, the limb contralateral to the last site should be used.

46. B. Distracting them with a role play.

Distraction is one way to take samples from pediatric patients. Others include anesthetic creams or ointments to numb the area. You might also need the help of their caregiver or parents to hold them steady.

47. D All of the above.

Butterfly/winged infusion sets are useful in pediatric or elderly patients or generally small veins.

48. B. Dermal puncture.

A dermal puncture is a phlebotomy procedure that is performed when a venipuncture might not be possible or when just a little sample of blood is required.

49. B. 2.0mm.

According to the AAP (American Academy of Pediatrics), heel punctures should not exceed a depth of 2.0 mm in infants.

50. C. 3rd finger.

In older children and adults, the distal portion of the 3rd or 4th finger is typically used.

51. D. All of the above.

Sites used - veins in forearm preferred, heel of the medial and lateral aspect of the plantar surface of the foot in infants, the distal aspect of 3rd or 4th finger in adults.
Prewarming - done in dermal puncture to increase the flow of blood to the finger
Technique - needle inserted into a vein to draw blood, puncture made with a lancet for dermal puncture.

52. B. Lavender, tube with additives, tube without additives.

The order of draw for puncture specimen:
Lavender-colored tubes, tubes with additives present, and tubes with additives absent.

53. B. Povidone iodine.

Povidone-iodine is avoided for dermal puncture as it interferes with several results.

54. A. ESR.

A dermal puncture cannot be used for ESR tests due to the large volume of blood required for the test.

55. C. Petechiae.

Petechiae refers to tiny, flat red spots that appear on the skin after a venipuncture procedure. They are caused by capillary rupture that can result from the tourniquet being left on for too long.

56. C. Never recap used needles.

Avoid recapping needles as much as possible. This is the standard practice all over the world in order to prevent needlestick injury.

57. C. Thrombophlebitis.

Thrombophlebitis means that there is blood clot formation, and the vein is also inflamed. Both can be avoided by the application of adequate pressure after the procedure.

58. B. Medial and lateral regions of the plantar surface of the foot.

59. B. Established systems to ensure a service meets the specified requirement.

Quality Assurance refers to systems, methods, and protocols that are set in place to ensure that a product or service meets the expected or specified requirements. Quality control becomes non-negotiable with systems that rely heavily on human involvement.

60. D. Failure of serum-cell preparation.

Some of the common errors that happen after sample collection include inappropriate use of serum separator, failure of serum-cell separation, delays in sample processing, exposing some samples to light inappropriately, poor storage conditions, rimming clots from overexposure of sample to air, failure to invert immediately after collection.

61. B. During sample collection.

During sample collection: Errors that occur during the collection of the sample include prolonged tourniquet time, hemolysis, blood clot formation, inappropriate order of draw, tube inversion done inadequately or not done at all, poor technique in sample collection, delays in taking the complete sample, not taking enough sample for the test.

62. C. Wrap with aluminum foil.

Dark sample bottles cannot be used for collection as they are not industry standard. However, light-sensitive samples can be wrapped with aluminum foil to protect them from light.

63. C. Arterial blood gasses.

Cold specimens: Samples for tests, such as arterial blood gasses, lactic acid, ammonia, and ACTh, should all be immediately placed inside containers with ice packs or crushed ices, to keep them cold and immediately transported to the laboratory for processing.

64. D. Samples for direct Coombs test.

Some other samples require higher temperatures for storage and processing. An excellent example of this is the direct Coombs test which requires that samples are placed in prewarmed containers at a temperature of 37 - 38 degrees Celsius for the removal of serum or plasma.

65. A. Fasting glucose is compared to glucose 2hrs after a meal.

66. B. Cortisol.

Cortisol exhibits diurnal variation and its peak levels are attained early in the morning, with a steady decline throughout the day.

67. C. Blood cultures.

68. B. 30 mins before the first dose.

The trough-level samples are typically used to measure the lowest level of the concentration of the drug in the blood. This is usually just before the next dose is administered.

69. C. Transport to the lab immediately, samples are affected by temperature and passage of time.

Blood culture samples are taken to check for the presence and identity of microorganisms in the patient's blood. This is usually done when there is suspected septicemia. The test is usually carried out aseptically, with blood culture bottles. The test samples should be taken to the laboratory as soon as they are collected because the results are affected by temperature and the passage of time.

70. C. Heel.

Phenylketonuria (PKU) Test is carried out to screen for the presence of phenylalanine which is seen in the condition phenylketonuria. It is an inheritable disease and must be detected at birth to prevent complications later in life. The sample used for this test is a few drops of blood taken from the heel of the newborn.

71. B. Toxicology.

Toxicology is analyzed in the chemistry section. Tests in the hematology section include CBC, ESR, coagulation studies, reticulocyte count, peripheral blood film, sickle cell, etc.

72. A. APTT.

This refers to Activated Partial Thromboplastin Time, and it is used to test for all the factors involved in the intrinsic and common pathways. It does this by measuring the time it takes that particular sample to form a clot after exposure to calcium and a phospholipid emulsion. The normal reference range is 30 -40 seconds.

73. B. PT.

Prothrombin time measures the time it takes for blood to clot via the extrinsic pathway. Therefore, it measures the efficiency of the extrinsic and the common pathways. This test specifically requires the tube to be about 60 - 80% full because of the presence of citrate, which is the common anticoagulant used in the sample collection.

74. A. Chemical reactions.

Chemical reactions of substances with each other takes place in the chemical section.

75. D. All of the above.

Tests carried out in the chemistry section include electrophoresis, immunochemistry, toxicology, liver profile tests, etc.

76. C. ADT.

The liver profile test is composed of Alkaline Phosphatase (ALP), Alanine Transaminase (ALT), Aspartate Transaminase (AST), Gamma Glutamyl Transferase (GGT), and bilirubin (direct and total).

77. D. Earlobe.

A toxic screen would usually require blood or urine samples. They can also use saliva, hair, or sweat for the screening.

78. B. HIV, HEP B.

Hepatitis B, C, and HIV can be transmitted through needlestick injuries. Hepatitis A is more commonly transmitted through the feco-oral route.

79. D. Serology/immunology.

This section is also involved in investigating the chances of acceptance or rejection of a body part or organ in the case of a transplant.

80. A. Microbiology.

The microbiology section is involved with the identification and quantification of parasites, pathogens, and microorganisms in the specimen provided.

81. C. The body produces antibodies against its own organs.

Autoimmune disorders happen when the body produces antibodies against its own organs and tissues. Antibodies are produced by the body against foreign bodies as an act of immunity, the humoral immunity. Not all autoimmune disorders are characterized by hypopigmentation. When a recipient's body rejects transplanted tissue, it is called transplant rejection.

82. B. Disorders that weaken the immune system.

83. C. Microbiology.

Microbiology is heavily involved in hospital infection control because they perform a lot of culture and sensitivity tests, which show not only the type of organism but also the drugs or antibiotics that it is sensitive to.

84. C. Culture and sensitivity.

Culture and sensitivity would help to identify unknown organisms which might be responsible for the fever and are defying routine antibiotics.

85. D. Hair.

Hair is not routinely used in microbiology. Hair is more common in chemistry and toxicology tests, also in forensic laboratories.

86. C. Results can take a longer time.

Some cultures can take a longer time to cultivate. Hence, physicians might find other methods to get a diagnosis or begin treatment with broad-spectrum antibiotics.

87. C. Color.

Macroscopic examination of urine looks at the physical properties of urine, such as its color, smell, clarity, and specific gravity.

88. B. Hemoconcentration.

Hemoconcentration results because the tourniquet now impedes the blood flow and increases the concentration of the cells in that segment relative to the plasma. This can lead to incorrect results if a sample is taken from that site.

89. D. None of the above.

The tests performed on urine include urine microscopy, culture, and sensitivity, which detect the presence of bacteria, fungi, and other pathogens in urine, as well as the antibiotics that they are sensitive to.

90. A. Diabetes insipidus.

Diabetes insipidus is diagnosed by the water deprivation test and vasopressin test. Here the patient is asked to refrain from drinking water and the amount of urine is measured. A large volume of dilute urine is suggestive. The vasopressin test helps confirm whether it is cranial or nephrogenic diabetes insipidus.

91. C. 2001.

92. D. All of the above.

The NeedleStick Prevention Act was updated to reflect 4 major areas: exposure control plan, employee input, record keeping and change of definitions.

93. C. Patient confidentiality.

Information should only be disclosed on a need-to-know basis. That is, people who would not need the information for the direct or indirect care of the patient do not need to know about the condition of the patient. In this case, the cleaner had absolutely no reason to know about the condition of the patient since the patient was in a different ward.

94. A. Implied consent.

Implied consent is given by an action. For instance, in phlebotomy, a patient stretching out the arm.

95. A. Going ahead to perform a procedure without asepsis and causing infection to the patient.

Tort: Refers to the inappropriate or wrong action that a person performs, which causes injury to another person. In the clinic, these can be battery, invasion of privacy, defamation of character through written (libel), or slander (spoken form).

96. B. Good Samaritan Law.

The Good Samaritan Law protects healthcare personnel, allowing them to render any healthcare service within the scope of their training in an accident or sudden injury without the fear of being charged with negligence.

97. B. Patient suffered harm or injury because she did not give the expected level of care.

Negligence refers to the failure of a person who is supposed to give a specific level of care to a patient, resulting in harm or loss to the patient. It is the failure to perform the level of care that anyone with the level of training and in the same circumstances would give.

98. A. Duty, derelict, direct cause, damage.

99. D. Derelict.

100. C. As much as important to perform their role as a phlebotomist.

Information should only be disclosed on a need-to-know basis. That is, people who would not need the information for the direct or indirect care of the patient do not need to know about the condition of the patient.

101. A. Acquired and innate.

102. A. T and B-cell mediated.

Acquired immunity can be classified into cellular immunity (T-cell mediated) and Humoral (B-cell mediated) immunity.

103. D. Innate.

104. C. Innate immunity.

Innate immunity refers to the inborn ability of the body to resist infectious agents.

105. C. Lymphocyte.

Both types of acquired immunity (T-cell and B-cell immunity) are mediated by lymphocytes.

106. D. B and C.

Cellular immunity is the function of T lymphocytes which are processed in the thymus. It is the type of immune response that the body produces without the production of antibodies. Instead, there is macrophage activation and NK-cells (natural killer cells) production.

107. D. All of the above.

Humoral immunity is a function of the B lymphocytes (B-cells) which are processed in the liver in utero and bone marrow after birth. Humoral immunity is characterized by the production of antibodies in response to the presence of an antigen on the surface of a pathogenic cell. This antigen first binds to a specific receptor on the B-cell that stimulates the production of numerous plasma cells, which now secrete large quantities of antibody molecules.

108. B. Process of antibodies marking pathogenic cells.

Antibodies can mark pathogenic cells in a process called opsonization, so that phagocytic cells (e.g., neutrophils, macrophages) can locate and destroy them.

109. A. Vasoconstriction, platelet plug formation, blood coagulation.

110. A. ADP.

Platelets begin to secrete ADP and thromboxane A2 after adherence. These substances help to attract more platelets.

111. D. All of the above.

The coagulation cascade has three stages:
1. The formation of the prothrombin activator: This occurs via 2 pathways which are the intrinsic and extrinsic pathways.
2. The conversion of prothrombin into thrombin
3. The conversion of fibrinogen to fibrin.

112. D. Fibrinolysis.

Fibrinolysis is the breakdown and removal of the clot from the inside of the blood vessel.

113. A. Vasoconstriction in hemostasis is systemic.

In hemostasis, vasoconstriction is not systemic. It is local to where the injury has occurred and is usually limited to the arterioles and small arteries.

114. B. Facilitates adherence.

115. A. No, phlebotomy is a field and a discipline. Venipuncture is a procedure.

The major phlebotomy procedure is venipuncture. Some people equate venipuncture to phlebotomy, but that is not correct. Phlebotomy as a field is more than venipuncture. It also involves other forms of sample collection, such as fingerstick sampling and arterial blood collection. It also involves the care of samples collected, the labeling and other things involved.

116. C. Sclerosed veins.

Sclerosed veins are usually seen in patients taking chemotherapy. It refers to the hardening of veins, which makes them cordlike in nature.

117. D. Arm with IV fluid running.

In choosing phlebotomy sites, avoid the arm that has an IV because it would affect the results of the tests.

118. A. Gray top.

The gray top contains antiglycolytic agents, which aim to prevent the breakdown of glucose and the sample through different mechanisms. It usually contains sodium fluoride oxalate or lithium. This bottle is typically used in the collection of fasting blood sugar, lactic acid, and glucose tolerance tests.

119. C. Green top.

120. A. SPS.

The yellow top tube is a sterile tube that usually contains SPS (sodium polyanethol sulfonate). It is used in taking samples for culture. It should be inverted 8 times after sample collection.

121. C. To ensure the patient gets well soon.

Infection control and safety procedures are not designed for the patient's speedy recovery but rather to reduce the risk of transmission of infectious agents and to ensure the safety of healthcare workers.

122. D. Disease-causing microorganisms.

Agents are the microorganisms responsible for causing infections.

123. C. Ensuring the patient wears the right personal protective equipment before phlebotomy.

124. A. Utilize transmission-based precautions with standard precautions.

Transmission-based precautions are used when a patient is suspected of or has been diagnosed with an infectious agent. They are tailored precautions that must accompany standard precautions.

125. D. None of the above.

Standard precautionary measures must be used at all times, irrespective of what is known or not known about the patient.

126. B. The phlebotomist technician putting on personal protective equipment.

Wearing personal protective equipment is how phlebotomist technicians can protect themselves from infectious agents.

127. B. Mode of transmission.

The droplet is one of the recognized five modes of transmission.

128. C. Susceptible host.

The microorganism leaves the reservoir through the portal of exit and uses the portal of entry to enter into a new host.

129. A. A host is a potential reservoir.

Once an individual is infected and becomes a new host, they become a potential reservoir through which infectious agents can be transmitted to others.

130. C. Agent ---> Mode of transmission ---> Susceptible host.

131. A. 5.

There are five modes of transmission.

132. D. Portal of exit, portal of entry.

The alimentary canal is an example of the portal of exit through which infectious agents leave a reservoir, and broken skin is an example of the portal of entry through which infectious agents enter the susceptible host.

133. B. Standard precautions.

Standard precautions in phlebotomy or any other healthcare practice are the precautions and routine activities that must be carried out in order to achieve a basic level of infection prevention and control.

134. B. All humans potentially harbor infectious agents.

Standard precautions are important because all living organisms and especially humans, potentially harbor infectious agents. These precautions will provide basic protection against any potential infection.

135. C. Use of respirators.

Using respirators is a transmission-based precaution that is done only when the patient is diagnosed or suspected to be infected with an airborne infectious agent.

136. D. Medical asepsis.

137. A. 1:10.

138. B. False.

Disinfectants are used on medical equipment, but not on human skin since they contain powerful chemicals that can irritate the skin and mucous membranes.

139. C. All of the above.

They are all examples of personal protective equipment used as a barrier protection against infectious agents.

140. D. Left uncapped after use and placed in a puncture-proof container.

Needles and other sharp objects used should be disposed of in puncture-proof containers and left uncapped.

141. B. Standard precautions alone will not suffice.

Transmission-based precautions are the infection prevention and control measures that are used when standard precautions alone will not suffice to prevent the spread of an infectious agent.

142. B. 3.
There are three distinct categories of transmission-based precautions.

143. D. None of the above.

144. B. Puncture-proof containers.

145. A. Properly labeling waste containers.

Waste containers should be properly labeled. Used needles should be left uncapped when they are being disposed of.

146. C. Sterilizing used equipment using steam.

147. A. Wastes that are potentially contaminated with infectious agents.

Biohazardous wastes are contaminated materials that, when not properly disposed of, can pose a new risk of infection to anyone who may come in contact with them.

148. C. Chemicals.

Chemicals that have not been contaminated with infectious agents are not considered biohazardous waste.

149. B. Respirators.

Respirators do not serve to protect the eyes.

150. A. They are strictly transmission-based precautions.

Barrier protection PPE can be both standard and transmission-based precautions. Most of them are, however, part of standard precautionary measures.

Anatomy and Physiology for Phlebotomists

Welcome to "Anatomy and Physiology for Phlebotomists." If you've found your way here, it's because you're ready to deepen your understanding and refine your skills in the fascinating world of phlebotomy. Following the success of "NHA Phlebotomy Exam Prep," this guide is designed to take you further into the essential anatomy and physiology knowledge that underpins our practice.

Purpose of This Guide

This book is more than just a collection of facts; it's a journey into the heart (quite literally!) of what makes phlebotomy such a vital part of healthcare. We'll explore the intricacies of the human body, focusing on how understanding anatomy and physiology enhances your capabilities as a phlebotomist. From the pulsing corridors of the cardiovascular system to the delicate dance of blood cells, we'll delve into the wonders that you encounter daily in your profession.

What Sets This Book Apart

I've tailored this guide to be straightforward and direct, stripping away the complex jargon without sacrificing the depth of information. Through vivid examples, real-world applications, and engaging case studies, we'll connect theory with the hands-on experiences that shape your career. My aim is to make learning both enjoyable and highly practical.

Scope of the Guide

Our focus will be on the systems most relevant to phlebotomy, especially the cardiovascular system. You'll learn about the journey of blood through the heart, the nuances of arteries, veins, and capillaries, and the fascinating interplay between pulse and blood pressure. While some aspects of anatomy and physiology are outside our scope, rest assured that what you find here will be immediately applicable to your work.

A Story of Challenge and Triumph

Let me share a story from my early days in phlebotomy. Like many, I faced challenges — tricky veins, anxious patients, and the pressure of getting it right. There was one particular day when everything that could go wrong did. But amidst that chaos, I learned an invaluable lesson: perseverance and a deep understanding of the human body turn challenges into victories. This incident didn't just make me a better phlebotomist; it reminded me of why we do what we do.

Inspiration for Your Journey

If you're just starting in phlebotomy, remember that every expert was once a beginner. This field is not just about skill but also about passion and the commitment to making a difference. Through this guide, I hope to inspire you to embrace each learning opportunity with enthusiasm and optimism.

How to Use This Guide

To get the most from this book, I recommend combining your reading with practical experiences. Reflect on the cases and analogies presented here and relate them to your daily tasks. This approach will solidify your understanding and enhance your skills.

Embracing the Journey Ahead

As you turn these pages, remember that you're not just learning; you're becoming an integral part of a community dedicated to care and compassion. Your journey through this book is a step towards excellence in your field. Approach it with an open mind, a curious heart, and the confidence that you can master its content.

Welcome to the next chapter of your phlebotomy career. Let's begin.

Chapter 1: The Circulatory System

Welcome to the first chapter of your advanced journey in phlebotomy. In this chapter, we delve into the circulatory system, the cornerstone of your daily work as a phlebotomist. Understanding this system is crucial, extending far beyond the mechanics of where to draw blood. It's about grasping the profound 'why' and 'how' of the body's most intricate transportation network.

At the heart of the circulatory system lies, quite literally, the heart. This remarkable muscular organ orchestrates the flow of life throughout your body. Functioning tirelessly, it pumps with a steady rhythm that begins before birth and continues until life's final moment. The heart is a dual-chambered powerhouse: the right side directs deoxygenated blood to the lungs for oxygenation, while the left side propels oxygen-rich blood to nourish the rest of the body. This efficient division ensures that every cell in the body receives the oxygen and nutrients it crucially needs.

Emerging from the heart is an intricate web of vessels – arteries, veins, and capillaries. Arteries, strong and elastic, carry blood away from the heart, while veins, more pliant and thinner, guide it back. The capillaries, delicate and prolific, are the sites of essential exchange: here, oxygen and nutrients are delivered to cells, and waste products are collected for removal. As a phlebotomist, your intimate knowledge of these vessels is not just technical; it's almost personal. It guides your hand during venipuncture, influencing where and how you draw blood.

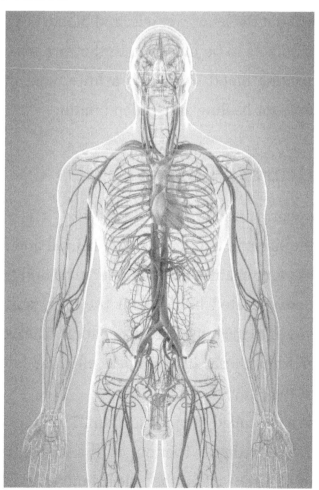

Blood, the medium in which you work daily, is a remarkable fluid. It's more than just cells in plasma; it's the body's primary means of internal communication. Carrying cells, nutrients, hormones, and waste, blood is the river of life that connects every part of the human organism. When you draw blood, you're accessing this essential system, gaining insights into the health and functioning of the body.

The practical application of this knowledge in phlebotomy cannot be overstated. Each element of the circulatory system plays a crucial role in your work. From selecting the appropriate vein for venipuncture to understanding the implications of the blood tests you perform, your expertise in the anatomy and physiology of the circulatory system is fundamental. It informs your technique, guides your decision-making, and enhances the care you provide to your patients.

As we explore the circulatory system in this chapter, remember that each piece of information, each detail about the heart, vessels, and blood, is a tool in your professional arsenal. These are not just facts to be memorized; they are insights to be applied. They are what transform a routine blood draw into a life-saving procedure, a moment of anxiety into an opportunity for healing and understanding.

Anatomy of the Heart and Blood Vessels

The heart, your field's central organ, is as complex as it is vital. Structurally, it's a muscular organ about the size of a fist, located just behind and slightly to the left of the breastbone. The heart has four chambers: two upper atria and two lower ventricles. The right atrium receives deoxygenated blood from the body and pumps it to the right ventricle, which then sends it to the lungs for oxygenation. The oxygen-rich blood returns to the left atrium, and from there, it's pumped into the left ventricle, which then distributes it throughout the body.

Surrounding the heart is a sac called the pericardium. This double-walled sac contains a small amount of fluid that reduces friction as the heart beats. The heart's walls themselves are made up of three layers: the epicardium (outer layer), the myocardium (the thick, muscular middle layer), and the endocardium (the inner layer).

The heart's function is regulated by an electrical system, which ensures that it beats in a coordinated and effective rhythm. This system includes the sinoatrial node, the heart's natural pacemaker, and the atrioventricular node, which regulates the impulses between the atria and ventricles.

Now, let's turn our attention to the blood vessels. The vessels are the highways of the circulatory system, transporting blood to every part of the body. They are categorized into three major types: arteries, veins, and capillaries.

- **Arteries:** These vessels carry blood away from the heart. The largest artery, the aorta, branches into smaller arteries, which then branch into even smaller arteries and arterioles throughout the body. Arterial walls are thick and elastic, allowing them to withstand the high pressure of blood pumped from the heart.

- **Veins:** Veins carry blood back to the heart. Unlike arteries, veins have thinner walls and less muscle tissue. They often have valves that prevent blood from flowing backward. The largest veins in the body are the superior and inferior vena cavae, which carry blood back to the right atrium of the heart.

- **Capillaries:** These are the smallest blood vessels and are where the exchange of oxygen, nutrients, carbon dioxide, and waste products occurs. Capillaries connect the arterial and venous systems. Their walls are just one cell thick, allowing for easy exchange between the blood and the tissues.

Understanding the anatomy of the heart and blood vessels is more than academic knowledge; it's a crucial part of your toolkit as a phlebotomist. This understanding guides your technique, informs your interactions with patients, and underpins the critical tests and treatments that rely on your expertise.

Venipuncture Sites and Their Anatomy

Venipuncture, the act of drawing blood, is a skill that balances anatomical knowledge with practical expertise. In my years of experience, I've come to understand that each venipuncture site has its unique characteristics and challenges. Let's explore some of the most common venipuncture sites and delve into their anatomy, accompanied by real-life examples and case studies.

1. The Median Cubital Vein: The Go-To Vein

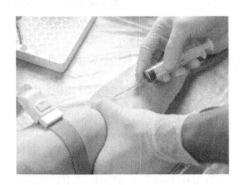

The median cubital vein, located in the antecubital fossa (the front of the elbow), is often the first choice for venipuncture. It's generally well anchored and less painful for patients when punctured. In my early days as a phlebotomist, I learned its value during a challenging blood draw on an elderly patient. The patient's skin was fragile, and their veins were difficult to palpate. However, the median cubital vein, being relatively stable and superficial, provided a successful draw. This experience taught me the importance of knowing your primary sites and their advantages.

2. The Cephalic Vein: The Alternative Choice

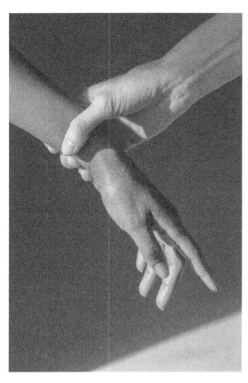

Situated along the lateral aspect of the arm, the cephalic vein can be more challenging due to its tendency to roll. I recall a particularly memorable case involving a bodybuilder with difficult-to-locate veins due to well-developed musculature. The cephalic vein, though less prominent, was the only viable option. Careful anchoring and a steady hand were crucial for a successful draw. This instance highlighted the importance of having backup sites and the skill to adapt to various patient anatomies.

3. The Basilic Vein: The Last Resort

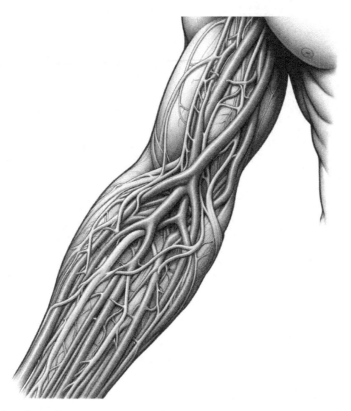

The basilic vein runs along the medial aspect of the arm and is often larger than other veins. However, it's close to nerves and arteries, making it a less preferred site. I remember a case where a patient with chronic illnesses had most of their accessible veins collapsed or scarred, except for the basilic vein. Despite the risks, it was the only option for venipuncture. The procedure required utmost precision to avoid complications. This experience underscored the need for thorough anatomical knowledge and careful consideration of risks in venipuncture.

4. Hand Veins: When Others Are Not Viable

Veins in the hand are usually smaller and can be more painful for the patient. However, they are sometimes the only accessible sites, especially in patients with a history of intravenous drug use or those who have undergone multiple medical procedures. In one case, a patient with severe dehydration presented a challenge as the typical venipuncture sites were not viable. The dorsal hand veins, though less comfortable, allowed for a successful blood collection. This scenario was a stark reminder of the need to be versatile and patient-focused in approach.

5. Pediatric and Geriatric Considerations

Working with pediatric and geriatric populations requires additional care. In children, the veins are smaller, and the experience can be frightening. A gentle approach and distraction techniques can be as important as technical skill. Similarly, in the elderly, veins can be fragile and prone to bruising. In both cases, choosing the right site and technique is crucial for patient comfort and successful venipuncture.

In Practice: Combining Knowledge with Empathy

Each venipuncture site has its peculiarities, and mastering them comes with experience and practice. But beyond the technical skill, it's the ability to empathize with patients, to understand their fears and discomforts, that truly makes a skilled phlebotomist. Balancing anatomical knowledge with a compassionate approach is what transforms a routine procedure into a positive experience for the patient.

Blood Components and Their Functions: An In-Depth Exploration

Blood, a vital fluid in the human body, is more than just a transporter of oxygen and nutrients. It is a complex system comprising various components, each with unique and essential functions. Understanding these components in detail is crucial for phlebotomists, as it enhances our ability to interpret laboratory results and communicate effectively with both healthcare teams and patients.

1. Red Blood Cells (Erythrocytes): The Oxygen Carriers

Red blood cells (RBCs) are the most numerous cells in blood. Their primary role is the transportation of oxygen from the lungs to the body's tissues and returning carbon dioxide from the tissues back to the lungs. RBCs are uniquely structured for this task; they are biconcave discs, which increases their surface area for oxygen absorption and release. The key to their function is hemoglobin, a complex protein that can bind oxygen and carbon dioxide. Hemoglobin not only transports gases but also imparts the red color to the blood.

Abnormalities in RBCs can lead to various clinical conditions. For example, in anemia, there is a deficiency in RBCs or hemoglobin, leading to reduced oxygen transport and resulting in fatigue and weakness. Conversely, in polycythemia, an excess of RBCs can increase blood viscosity, potentially leading to clotting problems.

2. White Blood Cells (Leukocytes): The Immune Defenders

White blood cells are the cornerstone of the body's immune system. They are fewer in number compared to RBCs but play a vital role in defending the body against infections, inflammation, and allergens. Leukocytes are classified into five main types, each with distinct functions:

- **Neutrophils**: The most abundant type of WBCs, crucial for combating bacterial infections.
- **Lymphocytes**: These cells are vital for immune response, including the production of antibodies (B cells) and cell-mediated immunity (T cells).
- **Monocytes**: They are the largest type of WBCs, important for phagocytosis (engulfing and digesting cellular debris and pathogens).
- **Eosinophils**: These cells are primarily involved in allergic reactions and fighting parasitic infections.
- **Basophils**: They are involved in inflammatory reactions and release histamine.

Elevated or decreased levels of WBCs can indicate various health conditions. For instance, leukopenia (low WBC count) can signify a compromised immune system, whereas leukocytosis (high WBC count) may indicate an ongoing infection or inflammation.

3. Platelets (Thrombocytes): The Clotting Specialists

Platelets, or thrombocytes, are tiny cell fragments crucial for blood clotting and wound healing. They are produced in the bone marrow and circulate in the blood, acting rapidly in response to bleeding. Upon encountering a damaged blood vessel, platelets adhere to the site and aggregate to form a plug, a process augmented by various clotting factors in plasma. This platelet plug is the first step in the complex process of blood clotting, which ultimately leads to the formation of a stable clot.

Thrombocytopenia (low platelet count) can lead to excessive bleeding, while thrombocytosis (high platelet count) may increase the risk of clot formation, potentially leading to conditions like stroke or heart attack.

4. Plasma: The Liquid Matrix

Plasma is the yellowish liquid component of blood, constituting about 55% of its total volume. It is composed primarily of water (about 90%), but also contains proteins (like albumin, globulins, and fibrinogen), electrolytes, nutrients, hormones, carbon dioxide, and waste products. Plasma serves several functions:

- **Transport Medium**: It carries cells, nutrients, waste products, hormones, and proteins throughout the body.
- **Regulatory Functions**: Plasma helps maintain blood pressure and volume and plays a critical role in thermoregulation.
- **Immune Functions**: It contains antibodies and other proteins essential for immune responses.

5. Serum: The Clot-Free Plasma

When blood clots, the liquid that remains is called serum. Serum is similar to plasma but lacks clotting factors. It is used in various diagnostic tests, especially those related to immune response, as it contains antibodies.

Interpreting Blood Tests in Phlebotomy

Each component of blood has specific implications in clinical diagnostics. For instance, a Complete Blood Count (CBC) provides a comprehensive overview of the cellular components, while biochemical tests on plasma or serum can assess metabolic functions, organ health, electrolyte balance, and more. As phlebotomists, understanding these components allows us to appreciate the significance of each blood test and the impact of their results on patient care.

Chapter 2: The Nervous System and Patient Care

As we venture into the realm of the nervous system in this chapter, we unravel its significant role in phlebotomy, particularly in the context of patient care. The nervous system, an intricate and vast network of neurons and pathways, forms the core of our interactions and experiences. In phlebotomy, understanding its nuances is not just about the science; it's about enhancing the patient experience and providing compassionate care.

The nervous system is essentially the body's command center, comprising the central nervous system (CNS) — the brain and spinal cord — and the peripheral nervous system (PNS), which includes all other neural elements. The CNS processes information and triggers responses, while the PNS connects the CNS to the rest of the body. The brain, a marvel in itself, interprets sensory information and governs emotions, while the spinal cord serves as the crucial conduit for transmitting signals between the brain and the body. When we delve deeper, we find the peripheral nervous system split into the somatic and autonomic systems. The somatic system oversees voluntary movements, and the autonomic system, split into sympathetic and parasympathetic branches, manages involuntary functions. The sympathetic system gears the body up for 'fight or flight,' and the parasympathetic system calms it down, encouraging 'rest and digest' responses.

In the context of phlebotomy, this knowledge is invaluable. Our patients' reactions, be it fear, anxiety, or even physical responses like a fluttering heart or sweating palms, are rooted in the workings of the nervous system. For instance, pain perception, a significant concern in venipuncture, is a complex interplay of sensory and emotional signals governed by the nervous system. Similarly, stress and anxiety trigger a symphony of reactions orchestrated by the sympathetic nervous system.

This understanding shapes our approach to patient care. Effective communication, for instance, isn't just about giving instructions; it's about engaging the patient in a way that activates their parasympathetic response, fostering calm and comfort. Similarly, distraction techniques do more than divert attention; they modulate the patient's sensory processing, reducing pain perception.

I've seen the power of these insights in action. In one memorable encounter, a patient with a deep-seated fear of needles was on the verge of a vasovagal response. Recognizing the signs early, I employed gentle conversation and a calming presence, which helped the patient relax, averting a fainting spell. In another instance, a patient with dementia required a different approach. Their altered neurological state made standard communication ineffective. By adapting my approach and involving their caregiver, we created an environment that was safe and reassuring, facilitating a successful venipuncture.

In these experiences lies the essence of phlebotomy. It's not just about drawing blood; it's about understanding the human being behind the procedure. The nervous system, in all its complexity, offers a window into our patients' experiences. By aligning our practices with this understanding, we not only enhance our technical skills but also elevate the level of compassion and empathy in our care.

Basics of the Nervous System: Structure and Function

The journey into the nervous system begins with an exploration of its structure and function. The nervous system, an elaborate and sophisticated network, is the epicenter of all bodily functions, sensations, and reactions. It's composed of two primary parts: the central nervous system (CNS) and the peripheral nervous system (PNS).

The CNS, consisting of the brain and spinal cord, is akin to a master control room. The brain, a marvel of nature, processes sensory information, orchestrates responses, and is the seat of our thoughts, emotions, and memories. Each part of the brain has a specialized role, from the frontal lobes responsible for reasoning and planning to the occipital lobes that interpret visual cues. The spinal cord, extending from the brain, is the major conduit for transmitting information between the brain and the rest of the body. It's not merely a messenger; it also processes reflexes and plays a role in many basic bodily functions.

The PNS extends the reach of the CNS to the rest of the body. It is divided into the somatic nervous system, which governs voluntary muscle movements and transmits sensory information to the CNS, and the autonomic nervous system, which controls involuntary bodily functions. The autonomic system is further divided into the sympathetic and parasympathetic systems, balancing the body's response to stress and relaxation.

Understanding the structure and function of the nervous system is vital, as it underpins every aspect of phlebotomy practice, from patient interactions to the interpretation of physiological responses during procedures.

Pain Perception and Stress Response During Venipuncture

Pain perception and the stress response during venipuncture are directly influenced by the nervous system. Pain, a complex and subjective experience, involves not just the physical sensation but also the emotional and psychological response to it. When a needle pierces the skin during venipuncture, nerve endings transmit signals through the spinal cord to the brain, which interprets these signals as pain. This process is influenced by various factors, including the patient's mental state, past experiences, and the context of the procedure.

The stress response, orchestrated by the sympathetic nervous system, is an automatic reaction to what the body perceives as a threat — in this case, the needle. This response triggers a cascade of physiological changes: the heart rate increases, blood pressure rises, and muscles tense. This 'fight or flight' response is an evolutionary mechanism, but in a clinical setting, it can create challenges for both the patient and the phlebotomist.

As phlebotomists, understanding these responses helps in mitigating pain and stress during venipuncture. Techniques like controlled breathing, proper positioning, and gentle technique can significantly reduce pain perception. Moreover, recognizing the signs of stress and responding with reassurance and empathy can help in calming anxious patients.

Communicating with Patients: Techniques for Anxiety Reduction

Effective communication is a cornerstone of patient care, particularly in reducing anxiety during venipuncture. The way we interact with patients can significantly influence their experience and response to the procedure. Communication in this context goes beyond words; it encompasses body language, tone of voice, and overall demeanor.

One effective technique is active listening. By attentively listening to patients' concerns and validating their feelings, we establish a rapport and trust. This connection can significantly alleviate anxiety. Another approach is the use of clear, simple explanations about the procedure. Understanding what to expect can demystify the process and reduce fear of the unknown.

Distraction techniques, such as engaging in light conversation or using visual or auditory distractions, can also be effective. These methods help shift the patient's focus away from the procedure, reducing pain perception and anxiety.

Lastly, demonstrating empathy and understanding is key. Acknowledging a patient's fear and offering reassurance can transform a potentially stressful experience into a more positive one. It's about creating an environment where patients feel heard, respected, and cared for.

In conclusion, these in-depth explorations of the nervous system's structure and function, pain perception and stress response during venipuncture, and techniques for effective patient communication provide a comprehensive understanding of the crucial role the nervous system plays in phlebotomy. This knowledge empowers phlebotomists to enhance patient care, making each interaction not just a medical procedure, but a compassionate, patient-centric experience.

Chapter 3: Blood Physiology and Sampling

Embark on an enriching journey into the realm of blood physiology and sampling, a chapter that offers a fresh perspective and deeper insights, distinct from what we've discussed so far. Here, we'll explore the subtleties of blood's composition and delve into the nuances of factors affecting blood tests, all while emphasizing the paramount importance of safety protocols in blood sampling.

Unique Aspects of Blood Composition

Diving deeper into blood's composition, we find a world teeming with life and activity. Beyond the basic understanding of red and white blood cells, and platelets, there's a myriad of functions each component performs. The RBCs, for instance, do more than just transport oxygen; they also play a role in regulating blood pH. WBCs, in their diversity, form a sophisticated defense network, each type specialized for specific pathogens. Platelets, often overlooked, are not just for clotting; they release growth factors that aid in healing. And plasma, the fluid matrix, is a treasure trove of nutrients, hormones, and proteins, each with a unique role in maintaining homeostasis.

Intricate Factors Influencing Blood Tests

When considering factors that affect blood tests, we move beyond the common culprits of hemolysis, fasting, and medication. For instance, the patient's hydration status can significantly alter certain test results, such as electrolyte levels and kidney function tests. Circadian rhythms, too, play a part – some blood components vary in concentration throughout the day. Even the patient's posture during blood draw – sitting or lying down – can influence the results. These subtleties make our role in preparing the patient and interpreting the results all the more critical.

Advanced Safety Protocols in Blood Sampling

Safety in blood sampling is a multifaceted endeavor. It's not just about wearing gloves or disposing of needles properly; it's about creating a safe environment. This includes meticulous attention to patient comfort and privacy, ensuring a calm and reassuring atmosphere during the draw. It's about being vigilant for signs of patient distress or adverse reactions, and being prepared to act swiftly and appropriately. Furthermore, maintaining the integrity of the sample through proper handling, storage, and transport is crucial – this ensures that the patient's journey through the testing process yields accurate and useful results.

In this chapter, we've taken a deeper, more nuanced look at the essentials of blood physiology and the art of blood sampling. This knowledge not only enhances our technical skills but also enriches our understanding of the profound impact our work has on patient care and medical diagnostics. As phlebotomists, we're not just practitioners of a medical procedure; we're integral players in the broader narrative of healthcare, where every blood sample tells a story and holds the key to understanding a patient's health. Let's carry this responsibility with pride and diligence, ever striving for excellence in our field.

Chapter 4: Special Populations in Phlebotomy

Navigating the challenges of phlebotomy in special populations requires a blend of technical skill, adaptability, and profound empathy. In this chapter, we delve into the world of pediatric and elderly patients, as well as individuals with special needs, offering insights and practical advice drawn from real-life experiences.

Pediatric Phlebotomy: Techniques and Considerations

Pediatric phlebotomy is a delicate balance between clinical proficiency and compassionate care. The fear and anxiety associated with needles are often magnified in young patients. Early in my career, I encountered a five-year-old girl terrified of needles. Her previous experiences had been traumatic, and she was visibly distressed. The approach here was twofold: technical precision and psychological comfort. Using a smaller butterfly needle, I ensured minimal discomfort. Simultaneously, I engaged her with a story, diverting her attention. The process was smooth, and her relieved smile at the end was profoundly rewarding.

When working with children, it's crucial to establish trust. This can involve explaining the procedure in simple terms, using distraction techniques like storytelling, or employing visual aids. Creating a child-friendly environment also helps – a room with colorful posters or a selection of toys can make a significant difference in a child's comfort level.

Phlebotomy in Elderly Patients: Vascular and Skin Considerations

Elderly patients often present with their unique set of challenges. I recall an 80-year-old patient with extremely fragile skin and prominent but fragile veins. The key was to use the lightest touch possible. I selected the most visible vein, applied the tourniquet gently, and used a smaller gauge needle to minimize trauma. Communication was also vital – I kept the patient informed throughout the process, which helped ease his anxiety.

In such cases, it's essential to take extra care with vein selection and to be mindful of the patient's comfort throughout the procedure. Elderly patients' skin requires careful handling to prevent bruising or tearing. Using a warm compress can sometimes make the veins more prominent and easier to access.

Adapting Techniques for Patients with Special Needs

Patients with special needs require a tailored approach. I remember working with a patient who had a severe physical disability, making the standard sitting position for venipuncture impractical. We had to adapt by using a specialized chair and ensuring that he was comfortable and stable throughout the procedure.

For patients with cognitive disabilities, patience and clear communication are key. Simplifying explanations and involving caregivers when necessary can greatly aid the process. For non-verbal patients, observing non-verbal cues becomes crucial to gauge their comfort and consent.

In all these scenarios, the common thread is the need for empathy and adaptability. Understanding the unique challenges each patient faces and adapting our approach accordingly is not just a professional requirement; it's a moral imperative.

The essence of phlebotomy in special populations lies in recognizing and respecting the diversity of patient needs. It's about creating a safe and comfortable environment for everyone, regardless of age, physical, or cognitive abilities. This approach not only ensures procedural success but also fosters a sense of dignity and respect for our patients. As phlebotomists, we're not just technicians; we're caregivers, and the role we play in our patients' healthcare journey is both significant and deeply meaningful.

Chapter 5: Infection Control and Immune Response

Welcome to Chapter 5, where we delve into the crucial world of infection control and the marvels of the immune system. This chapter is not just about procedures and protocols; it's a journey through some of the most defining moments of my career as a phlebotomist, offering you insights and inspirations that I hope will guide and uplift you in your own journey.

The Frontline of Defense: Infection Control

Infection control in phlebotomy is not just about following guidelines; it's about being a guardian of health. I remember an incident early in my career when a minor oversight in sanitization protocol led to a nerve-wracking 48 hours, waiting to see if a patient would develop an infection. Thankfully, they didn't. But that experience imprinted on me the gravity of our responsibility. Since then, I've been meticulous about infection control, treating it as a sacred duty to my patients and myself.

In this section, we'll explore:

- Hand hygiene: the simple yet powerful tool in infection prevention.
- Personal protective equipment (PPE): your armor in the healthcare battlefield.
- Proper disposal of sharps and other biohazard materials: keeping the environment safe for everyone.
- Sanitization protocols: ensuring every step of the process is clean and secure.

Harnessing the Power of the Immune System

Understanding the immune response is like decoding a superpower within us. It's fascinating, complex, and absolutely crucial for a phlebotomist. I once had a patient with a compromised immune system, and drawing blood required extra precautions. The experience taught me the incredible resilience of the human body and the importance of our role in supporting it.

Here, we'll cover:

- The basics of the immune system: how this intricate network guards our health.
- Immunological tests: how your work as a phlebotomist contributes to life-saving diagnoses.
- Working with immunocompromised patients: the heightened care and empathy required.
- Vaccinations and phlebotomy: understanding your role in this critical aspect of healthcare.

Real-Life Heroes: Stories of Challenges and Triumph

This section is close to my heart. Here, I share stories of challenges I faced and how I overcame them. Like the time I had to draw blood from a patient with severe needle phobia. With patience, empathy, and a gentle technique, I turned a terrifying experience for them into a manageable one. It was a moment of profound learning and personal growth.

You'll find stories of:

- Navigating difficult blood draws: the technique, the patience, and the triumph.
- Communicating with patients: building trust in moments of vulnerability.
- Learning from mistakes: how each misstep is a stepping stone to mastery.
- The emotional rollercoaster: handling the highs and lows with grace and resilience.
- **Immune System Overview: Key Components**
- The immune system is a masterpiece of biological engineering, a silent guardian that tirelessly works to keep us safe from myriad threats. As a phlebotomist, appreciating the complexity and efficiency of this system can greatly enhance the care you provide. At the heart of the immune system are two key players: the innate and adaptive immune responses.
- The innate immune response is the body's first line of defense, acting rapidly against invaders. It includes physical barriers like skin and mucous membranes, as well as immune cells like neutrophils and macrophages. These cells are like the unsung heroes, always on the frontlines, ready to tackle pathogens. I recall a case where understanding the significance of an elevated neutrophil count helped identify an early infection in a patient, enabling prompt treatment.
- The adaptive immune system is more specialized and remembers past invaders. It involves lymphocytes, such as B cells and T cells. B cells produce antibodies, while T cells destroy infected cells. The beauty of this system is its memory – once exposed to a pathogen, it can swiftly respond to future encounters. This is the principle behind vaccinations, a crucial part of public health that we as phlebotomists support through blood tests for antibody levels.
- In this vast network, the spleen and lymph nodes act as command centers, orchestrating the immune response. Understanding these components not only

aids in our technical knowledge but also in empathizing with patients who have immune-related conditions.

- **Best Practices in Infection Control and Safety**
- Infection control is the cornerstone of safe phlebotomy practice. It's a commitment to patient safety and your own. The first step is always hand hygiene. Wash your hands thoroughly and frequently, and use hand sanitizer when washing isn't possible. This simple practice is powerful – I've seen it drastically reduce the risk of hospital-acquired infections.
- Personal protective equipment (PPE) is your armor. Always wear gloves, and if there's a risk of splashes, don a face shield or mask. Remember, changing gloves between patients isn't just a guideline, it's an act of respect for each individual's health.
- Needlestick injuries are a grim reality in our field. Always use safety-engineered devices and never recap needles. In my early days, I learned this the hard way when I suffered a needlestick injury. It was a stressful experience, waiting for test results, but it taught me to never let my guard down.
- Disposal of sharps and other biohazard materials is equally crucial. Use designated sharps containers and handle biohazard waste responsibly. Once, a colleague of mine overlooked this, leading to a minor outbreak of infection in our facility. It was a wake-up call for all of us about the importance of diligent disposal.
- Finally, stay up-to-date with vaccination protocols. As healthcare providers, we need to be protected to keep our patients safe. Regular training and refreshers on infection control can be life-saving.

Handling and disposing of contaminated materials is a critical aspect of maintaining a safe and hygienic healthcare environment. As a phlebotomist, I've learned that the way we manage these materials directly impacts not only our safety but also the safety of our patients and colleagues.

Understanding Contaminated Materials

Firstly, it's important to understand what constitutes contaminated material. In the realm of phlebotomy, this typically includes used needles, blood vials, gloves, gauze, or any other items that have come into contact with blood or bodily fluids. These materials are potentially infectious and require careful handling.

Effective Handling Techniques

When handling contaminated materials, always wear appropriate personal protective equipment (PPE), such as gloves and, if necessary, face protection. Never touch these materials with bare hands. For instance, after drawing blood, I always make sure to carefully remove the needle using a safety device and avoid touching any part that has come into contact with the patient's blood.

Proper Disposal Methods

1. **Sharps Disposal:** Needles and other sharps should be immediately disposed of in a designated sharps container. These containers are typically puncture-resistant and labeled for easy identification. It's crucial never to overfill sharps containers or try to force items into them, as this can lead to needlestick injuries. In my practice, we ensure that sharps containers are easily accessible and replaced regularly.

2. **Biohazard Waste:** Other contaminated materials, such as used gloves, gauze, or bandages, should be disposed of in biohazard waste bags. These bags are usually red or yellow and marked with a biohazard symbol. It's essential to seal these bags securely before disposing of them in the designated biohazard waste disposal area.

3. **Handling Spills:** In the event of a blood or bodily fluid spill, it's important to act quickly. Use appropriate absorbent materials and disinfectants, and always wear gloves and other necessary PPE. Once the spill is cleaned, dispose of any used cleaning materials as biohazard waste.

Personal Experience and Tips

In my years of experience, I've encountered a few incidents where proper disposal was overlooked, leading to safety hazards. One such instance was when a sharps container was overfilled, and a colleague suffered a needlestick injury. This incident reinforced the importance of timely and proper disposal.

Here are some additional tips from my experience:

- Regularly check the fill levels of sharps containers and biohazard waste bags.
- Educate all staff on the importance of proper disposal procedures.
- Report any safety hazards or incidents immediately to the appropriate department.
- Never rush when handling contaminated materials, as this increases the risk of accidents.

Integrating Knowledge into Practice

In phlebotomy, the integration of knowledge into practice is crucial for delivering high-quality patient care. This integration is not just about having theoretical knowledge; it's about applying that knowledge skillfully in real-world scenarios. Over the years, I've learned that the bridge between knowing and doing is built through experience, reflection, and a willingness to adapt.

One of the key areas where integration becomes vital is in understanding patient physiology. For instance, when drawing blood from a patient with dehydration, I apply my knowledge about the effects of dehydration on vein accessibility. This understanding guides me to choose the most appropriate technique and equipment for the procedure.

Another aspect is in the interpretation of test results. Understanding the implications of various blood tests allows me to be more empathetic towards patients and provide them with better care. For example, knowing the potential stress a diabetes patient might be experiencing before a fasting glucose test helps in offering them the right support and guidance.

Techniques for Effective Integration

- **Hands-on Practice:** There's no substitute for actual practice. Engaging in regular, hands-on procedures under supervision, initially, helps solidify theoretical knowledge.
- **Simulation Training:** Using simulation models or participating in role-play scenarios can be extremely helpful in preparing for real-life situations.

- **Reflective Practice:** After each procedure, take time to reflect on what went well and what could be improved. This reflection enhances learning and integration of new skills.
- **Peer Learning:** Observing and discussing techniques with experienced colleagues can provide valuable insights and practical tips.

Importance of Continuous Learning in Phlebotomy

Phlebotomy, like all healthcare fields, is ever-evolving. Continuous learning is vital to stay current with the latest techniques, technologies, and best practices. This ongoing education not only improves proficiency but also enhances patient safety and care quality.

For instance, staying updated with the latest advancements in needle technology and vein visualization tools can significantly improve the efficiency and comfort of blood draws. Similarly, understanding new guidelines on infection control, especially in the wake of global health crises like the COVID-19 pandemic, is crucial.

As you continue on this path, embrace the challenges and opportunities that come with being a phlebotomist. Remember the profound impact you can have on patients' lives. Your role is crucial, your skills are invaluable, and your capacity for growth is limitless.

Let this journey be one of continuous learning, skillful practice, and heartfelt empathy. Stand proud as a vital member of the healthcare team, and carry forward the legacy of excellence in phlebotomy. The path ahead is as rewarding as it is demanding, and each step you take is a testament to your dedication to this noble profession.

CONTACT THE AUTHOR

I always strive to make this guide as comprehensive and helpful as possible, but there's always room for improvement. If you have any questions, suggestions, or feedback, I would love to hear from you. Hearing your thoughts helps me understand what works, what doesn't, and what could be made better in future editions.

To make it easier for you to reach out, I have set up a dedicated email address:

✉ epicinkpublishing@gmail.com

Feel free to email me for:

- Clarifications on any topics covered in this book

- Suggestions for additional topics or improvements

- Feedback on your experience with the book

- Any other inquiries you may have

Your input is invaluable. I read every email and will do my best to respond in a timely manner.

Thank you once again for entrusting me with a part of your educational journey. I wish you all the best in your upcoming exam and future endeavors in the electrical field.

Best wishes

References

A. (2022, February 21). *Dermal Puncture and Capillary Blood Collection.* LabUniversity. https://labuniversity.org/dermal-puncture-and-capillary-blood-collection/

Aghoghovwia, B. (2022, November 28). *Veins of the upper limb.* Kenhub. https://www.kenhub.com/en/library/anatomy/veins-of-the-upper-limb

Arteries: What They Are, Anatomy & Function. (n.d.). Cleveland Clinic. https://my.clevelandclinic.org/health/body/22896-arteries#:~:text=Arteries%20distribute%20oxygen%2Drich%20blood,and%20hormones%20throughout%20your%20body.

Barbucci, R. (1998). Heparin-like New Molecules with Blood. *Elsevier EBooks,* 339–357. https://doi.org/10.1016/b978-044420524-7/50027-8

Biguria, J. F., MD. (n.d.). *Venous Drainage Anatomy: Overview, Microscopic Anatomy, Other Considerations.* https://emedicine.medscape.com/article/1899411-overview#a1

Black, C. M. (2014a). Anatomy and Physiology of the Lower-Extremity Deep and Superficial Veins. *Techniques in Vascular and Interventional Radiology, 17*(2), 68–73. https://doi.org/10.1053/j.tvir.2014.02.002

Black, C. M. (2014b). Anatomy and Physiology of the Lower-Extremity Deep and Superficial Veins. *Techniques in Vascular and Interventional Radiology, 17*(2), 68–73. https://doi.org/10.1053/j.tvir.2014.02.002

Blood Collection Procedure: Capillary» Pathology Laboratories» College of Medicine» University of Florida. (n.d.). https://pathlabs.ufl.edu/client-services/specimen-shipping/blood-collection-procedure-capillary/:~:text=Capillary%20punctures%20are%20not%20suitable,testing%20and%20most%20coagulation%20tests.

Bolton-Maggs, P. H. B., & Flavin, A. (2005). Epirubicin for breast cancer may cause considerable venous sclerosis. *BMJ, 331*(7520), 816. https://doi.org/10.1136/bmj.38574.659225.79

Collie, J. C., MD. (n.d.). *Cold Agglutinin Disease Workup: Approach Considerations, Complete Blood Cell Count and Peripheral Smear, Reticulocytes and Spherocytes.* https://emedicine.medscape.com/article/135327-workup

Crna, R. N. M. (2020a, January 13). *Bruising after a blood draw: What to know.* https://www.medicalnewstoday.com/articles/327464#:~:text=According%20to%20the%20World%20Health,weeks%20to%20fade%20and%20disappear.

Crna, R. N. M. (2020b, January 13). *Bruising after a blood draw: What to know.* https://www.medicalnewstoday.com/articles/327464#:~:text=According%20to%20the%20World%20Health,weeks%20to%20fade%20and%20disappear.

Deacon, B. J., & Abramowitz, J. S. (2006). Fear of needles and vasovagal reactions among phlebotomy patients. *Journal of Anxiety Disorders, 20*(7), 946–960. https://doi.org/10.1016/j.janxdis.2006.01.004

Diabetes Insipidus: Causes, Symptoms, Diagnosis & Treatment. (n.d.). Cleveland Clinic. https://my.clevelandclinic.org/health/diseases/16618-diabetes-insipidus

F., & F. (2021, January 13). *Basic Phlebotomy Principles.* PhlebotomyU. https://phlebotomyu.com/basic-phlebotomy-principles/#:~:text=After%20blood%20withdrawal%20has%20occurred,again%2C%20to%20protect%20against%20infections.

Faap, E. T. R. M. (n.d.). *Phenylketonuria (PKU): Practice Essentials, Background, Pathophysiology.* https://emedicine.medscape.com/article/947781-overview

Fcap, J. T. M. D. (n.d.). *Thrombin Time: Reference Range, Interpretation, Collection and Panels.* https://emedicine.medscape.com/article/2086278-overview

Fccp, E. C. M. (n.d.-a). *Bleeding Time: Reference Range, Interpretation, Collection and Panels.* https://emedicine.medscape.com/article/2085022-overview#a1

Fccp, E. C. M. (n.d.-b). *Bleeding Time: Reference Range, Interpretation, Collection and Panels.* https://emedicine.medscape.com/article/2085022-overview

González-López, M., MD. (n.d.-a). *Arterial Supply Anatomy: Overview, Gross Anatomy, Microscopic Anatomy.* https://emedicine.medscape.com/article/1898807-overview

González-López, M., MD. (n.d.-b). *Arterial Supply Anatomy: Overview, Gross Anatomy, Microscopic Anatomy.* https://emedicine.medscape.com/article/1898807-overview

Gupta, J. I., & Shea, M. J. (2023, March 15). *Biology of the Heart.* MSD Manual Consumer Version. https://www.msdmanuals.com/home/heart-and-blood-vessel-disorders/biology-of-the-heart-and-blood-vessels/biology-of-the-heart

Hammami, M. B., MD. (n.d.). *Partial Thromboplastin Time, Activated: Reference Range, Interpretation, Collection and Panels.* https://emedicine.medscape.com/article/2085837-overview#a2

Hashemi, R. (2015, January 1). *Erythrocyte Sedimentation Rate Measurement Using as a Rapid Alternative to the Westergren Method.* PubMed Central (PMC). https://www.ncbi.nlm.nih.gov/pmc/articles/PMC4614602/

How do health care providers diagnose phenylketonuria (PKU)? (2016, December 1). https://www.nichd.nih.gov/. https://www.nichd.nih.gov/health/topics/pku/conditioninfo/diagnosed

Kapoor, D. (2022, October 10). *Blog Title.* Virohan. https://www.virohan.com/blog/what-are-the-techniques-that-make-phlebotomy-efficient

Lago, C. L. D., Daniel, D., Lopes, F., & Cieslarova, Z. (2020). Electrophoresis. *Elsevier EBooks,* 499–523. https://doi.org/10.1016/b978-0-12-813266-1.00010-3

Lower limb: Anatomy study course | Kenhub. (n.d.). Kenhub. https://www.kenhub.com/en/start/lower-extremity

Lucchetti, L. (2022, November 10). *Understanding Chemotherapy Extravasation: Causes and Management.* Healthline. https://www.healthline.com/health/cancer/chemotherapy-extravasation#causes-and-risk-factors

McDiarmid, S. V. (2015). Special Considerations for Immunosuppression in Children. *Science Direct.* https://doi.org/10.1016/b978-1-4557-0268-8.00092-0

N. (2023, March 8). *Collecting a Specimen Sample: 3 Methods Examined.* https://www.neoteryx.com/microsampling-blog/the-best-way-to-collect-a-blood-sample-3-methods-examined

Needlestick safety and prevention act. (2001, April 1). PubMed. https://pubmed.ncbi.nlm.nih.gov/16902692/

News-Medical.net. (2019, February 27). *Hematology Tests.* https://www.news-medical.net/health/Hematology-Tests.aspx

NIOSH Needlestick Prevention Resource Shares Lessons Learned From Real-Life Programs | NIOSH | CDC. (n.d.). https://www.cdc.gov/niosh/updates/needleless.html#:~:text=Under%20the%20Needlestick%20Safety%20and,reduce%20the%20risk%20of%20needlesticks.

Phlebotomists: Occupational Outlook Handbook: U.S. Bureau of Labor Statistics. (2022, September 22). https://www.bls.gov/ooh/healthcare/phlebotomists.htm#tab-1

Post Blood Collection Hematoma Care Instructions. (n.d.). UK HealthCare. https://ukhealthcare.uky.edu/services/laboratory-services/hematoma-care

Prothrombin time test - Mayo Clinic. (2022, November 30). https://www.mayoclinic.org/tests-procedures/prothrombin-time/about/pac-20384661

TeachMeAnatomy. (2018, November 6). *Venous Drainage of the Upper Limb - Basilic - Cephalic - TeachMeAnatomy.* https://teachmeanatomy.info/upper-limb/vessels/veins/

Testing Situations When Capillary Blood Collection is Not Appropriate - LabCE.com, Laboratory Continuing Education. (n.d.).

https://www.labce.com/spg860124_testing_situations_when_capillary_blood_collect
ion.aspx

Thanassoulis, G., & Aziz, H. (2023, March 15). *Atherosclerosis*. MSD Manual Consumer Version. https://www.msdmanuals.com/home/heart-and-blood-vessel-disorders/atherosclerosis/atherosclerosis

The Dangers of Needle Recapping and How to Protect Yourself | Animal Care. (n.d.). https://animalcare.umich.edu/announcements/dangers-needle-recapping-and-how-protect-yourself#:~:text=Recapping%20needles%20is%20extremely%20dangerous,drugs%2C%20or%20infectious%20biological%20agents.

Tishkowski, K. (2022, May 8). *Erythrocyte Sedimentation Rate*. StatPearls - NCBI Bookshelf. https://www.ncbi.nlm.nih.gov/books/NBK557485/

Tuazon, S. A., MD. (n.d.). *Prothrombin Time: Reference Range, Interpretation, Collection and Panels*. https://emedicine.medscape.com/article/2086058-overview#a4

What to Know About Bruising After a Blood Draw. (2021, May 7). WebMD. https://www.webmd.com/a-to-z-guides/what-to-know-about-bruising-after-blood-draw

Winona Health. (2022, March 14). *Laboratory Departments and Overview*. https://www.winonahealth.org/health-care-providers-and-services/specialty-care-services/laboratory/laboratory-departments-and-overview/#:~:text=It%20is%20defined%20as%20the,and%20hormone%20tests%2C%20and%20PSA.

Made in United States
North Haven, CT
27 February 2024

49294150R00109